William Cullen
and the
Eighteenth Century Medical World

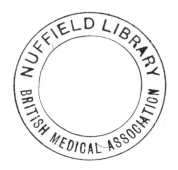

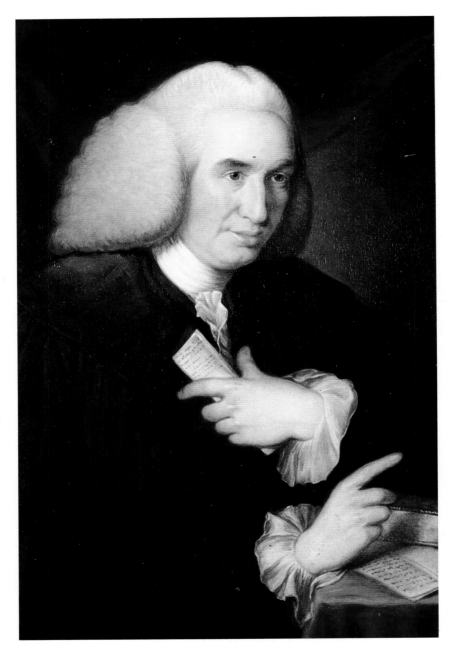

WILLIAM CULLEN
Age 58, 1768, after William Cochrane

William Cullen
and the
Eighteenth Century
Medical World

A bicentenary exhibition and symposium
arranged by the Royal College of Physicians
of Edinburgh in 1990

edited by

A. DOIG, J.P.S. FERGUSON, I.A. MILNE AND R. PASSMORE

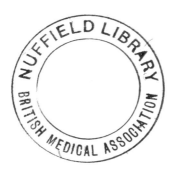

EDINBURGH UNIVERSITY PRESS

© Edinburgh University Press, 1993

Edinburgh University Press
22 George Square, Edinburgh

Typeset in Linotron Times Roman
by Photoprint, Torquay, and
printed in Great Britain by
The Alden Press, Oxford

A CIP record for this book is available
from the British Library

ISBN 0 7486 0302 6

Royal College of Physicians of Edinburgh
Publication no 62

Contents

Foreword

This book is a record of an exhibition and a symposium commemorating the two hundredth anniversary of the death of William Cullen in 1790. The exhibition and symposium were organised by the Royal College of Physicians in Edinburgh of which he was President from 1773 to 1775. The book has been published by the press of Edinburgh University where Cullen was successively professor of chemistry, of physiology and of medicine.

Papers in the symposium assess the contributions of Cullen to the theory and practice in his time of the three subjects that he taught. But this book, it is hoped, will interest others besides historians of science and medicine. William Cullen was a prominent figure among the personalities of the Scottish Enlightenment. He was a sociable and clubbable man. Adam Smith and David Hume were his intimate friends. Boswell invited him to meet Dr Johnson at a small supper party on their brief visit to Edinburgh.

Above all Cullen was a great teacher and, more than any other, was responsible for Edinburgh being the foremost medical school in the world of his day. He attracted many students from the American colonies and the medical schools and institutions founded by his pupils set the pattern of medicine in the United States.

The College will be delighted if this book introduces young men and women of the present day to an attractive member of the distinguished society that flourished two hundred years ago in Scotland and which had a great influence throughout the world.

JOHN RICHMOND
President, Royal College of Physicians of Edinburgh
January 10th 1991

Contributors

M. BARFOOT
Medical Archive Centre, Edinburgh University Library, George Square, Edinburgh, EH8 9LJ. U.K.

E.G. BUCKLEY
Royal College of General Practitioners, 12 Queen Street, Edinburgh, EH2 1JE. U.K.

W.F. BYNUM
Wellcome Institute for the History of Medicine, 183 Euston Road, London, NW1 2BP. U.K.

J.R.R. CHRISTIE
Department of Philosophy, Division of the History and Philosophy of Science, The University of Leeds, Leeds, LS2 9JT. U.K.

C. CLAYSON
Cockiesknowe, Lochmaben, Lockerbie, Dumfriesshire, DG11 1RL. U.K.

A. DOIG
Royal College of Physicians, 9 Queen Street, Edinburgh, EH2 1JQ, U.K.

R.L. EMERSON
Department of History, Faculty of Social Science, University of Western Ontario, London, Ontario, Canada, N6A 5C2

J.P.S. FERGUSON
Royal College of Physicians, 9 Queen Street, Edinburgh, EH2 1JQ, U.K.

R.E. KENDELL
University Department of Psychiatry, Royal Edinburgh Hospital, Morningside, Edinburgh, EH10 5HF.

D.C. MACARTHUR
Royal Medical Society, Students' Centre, 5/5 Bristo Square, Edinburgh, EH8 9AL, U.K.

I.A. MILNE
Royal College of Physicians, 9 Queen Street, Edinburgh, EH2 1JQ, U.K.

J.M. O'DONNELL
The College of Physicians of Philadelphia, 19 South Twenty-Second Street, Philadelphia, PA 19103, U.S.A.

R. PASSMORE
Royal College of Physicians, 9 Queen Street, Edinburgh, EH2 1JQ, U.K.

G.B. RISSE
Department of the History of Health Sciences, University of California, 533 Parnassus Avenue, San Francisco, CA 91413–0726, U.S.A.

Acknowledgements

We wish to thank the following institutions and individuals who granted us permission to display material in the exhibition and allowed us to illustrate many of the selected items in this volume:

City of Edinburgh Art Centre
College of Physicians of Philadelphia
Collection at Lennoxlove, the Duke of Hamilton
The Honourable Lord Cullen
Edinburgh City Libraries
Edinburgh University Library
Falkirk Museums
Glasgow Museums
Hamilton District Council
Hamilton District Museum
Heriot-Watt University, Edinburgh
Hunterian Art Gallery, University of Glasgow
Independence National Historical Park Collection, Philadelphia
Mrs P.M. Maxwell-Scott
Dr P.A.G. Monro
National Gallery of Scotland
National Library of Scotland
National Portrait Gallery, London
Royal College of Physicians of London
Royal College of Surgeons of Edinburgh
Royal Infirmary of Edinburgh
Royal Medical Society
Miss A. Scott-Plummer
Scottish National Portrait Gallery
University of Edinburgh

We are also indebted to Mr Jim Paul and Mr Harry Phillips of the Medical Illustration Service, University of Edinburgh, for photography, to Miss Allyson Bain for the design of display panels and Mr Tom Ewing for arranging publicity. We gratefully acknowledge the assistance of the following members of the staff of the College: Mr Iain Elliot, Mrs Norma Macdonald, Mr George Tait, Mrs Margaret Pringle, Miss Jennifer Heron, Mrs Marion Jack, Mrs Jenny Spencer, Mr Robert Wyse, Mr Andrew Duncan and Mr Michael Ellis. We thank Mrs Anne McCarthy for preparing the index. Astra Pharmaceuticals Limited generously defrayed the cost of publishing the illustrations. This bicentenary celebration owed much to the enthusiasm and active support of Dr John Richmond, President of the College.

Illustrations

The editors wish to thank the individuals and the institutions acknowledged in the captions for their kind permission to reproduce these illustrations.

A Chronology of the Life of William Cullen
1710–1790

1710	Born on April 15 at Hamilton, Lanarkshire where his father was a lawyer and factor to the Duke of Hamilton and his mother was a member of the Roberton family of Whistlebury
1726–9	Student at Glasgow University (Arts course in general studies) Apprentice surgeon apothecary to John Paisley of Glasgow
1729	Surgeon on a merchant ship to the West Indies
1730–1	Assistant apothecary to Mr Murray of Henrietta Street, London
1732–3	General practitioner, Shotts, Lanarkshire
1733–6	Further education, financed by small legacy General literature and philosophy (private study) Medical classes at Edinburgh University
1736–44	General practitioner/surgeon in Hamilton Also served in Hamilton as town councillor (1737–44) and magistrate (1738–41)
1740	Awarded degree of Doctor of Medicine, in Glasgow
1741	Married Anna Johnstone, daughter of the Reverend Robert Johnstone of Kilbarchan
1744	Moved to Glasgow. Set up as a practising physician and as an extramural medical teacher
1746–55	Lectures on medicine and physiology in the University of Glasgow

1747–9	President of the Faculty of Physicians and Surgeons of Glasgow
1747–50	Lectures on materia medica and botany in the University of Glasgow
1747–55	Lecturer in chemistry, University of Glasgow
1751–5	Professor of medicine, University of Glasgow
1755–66	Professor of chemistry and medicine, University of Edinburgh
1757–74	Lectures on clinical medicine in Edinburgh Royal Infirmary
1766–73	Professor of the institutes (theory) of medicine, University of Edinburgh
1768	Gave private course of lectures on vegetation and agriculture, published posthumously in 1796
1769	Joint professor of the institutes and the practice of medicine, University of Edinburgh *Synopsis nosologiae methodicae*
1772	*Lectures on the materia medica as delivered by William Cullen MD* (pirated edition published in London) *Lectures on the institutions of medicine, part 1, physiology*
1773–89	Sole professor of the practice of physic (medicine), University of Edinburgh
1773–90	First Physician to the King in Scotland
1773–5	President of the Royal College of Physicians of Edinburgh
1777–84	*First lines of the practice of physic* (4 volumes)
1777	Elected Fellow of the Royal Society of London
1778	Purchased Ormiston Hill Farm, at Kirknewton, Midlothian
1783	Founder member of the Royal Society of Edinburgh
1789	*A treatise of the materia medica* (2 volumes)
1790	Died in Edinburgh on February 5 and was interred at Kirknewton

THE EXHIBITION

The Cullen Bicentenary Exhibition

ANDREW DOIG, JOAN P.S. FERGUSON AND IAIN A. MILNE

This pictorial biography is based on the Bicentenary Exhibition which was open to the public in the New Library of the College from 18–25 August 1990. Commentaries on the 106 exhibits and 62 illustrations provide an introduction to the life of William Cullen and his influence on the development of medicine and science during the Scottish Enlightenment.

The opening sections deal with *Cullen's boyhood in Lanarkshire* and his period of *General practice in Hamilton* where he was assisted by William Hunter. At the *University of Glasgow* he gave lectures on chemistry, botany, materia medica and medicine. He became a professor at the same time as Adam Smith and was a founder of the Glasgow Medical School. Cullen's interests in *Chemistry and agriculture* gained him the patronage of Lord Kames and the Duke of Argyll who each had a decisive role in his appointment to the chair of chemistry in Edinburgh. He brought a new approach to *Infirmary and University teaching in Edinburgh* which enhanced the reputation of the medical school. *Cullen's influence on American medicine* stemmed largely from his friendship with Benjamin Franklin who sent him promising students, many of whom became pioneers in medical education in the New World. Cullen was *Mentor* to many men of distinction including Joseph Black, discoverer of carbon dioxide, William Withering of foxglove fame and John Rogerson, physician to Catherine the Great. He was an active supporter of the *Royal Medical Society* where students presented their dissertations and debated and his writings as a noted *Bibliophile and author* were standard texts in the medical world of his time.

Most of Cullen's professional and social activities in Edinburgh were within walking distance of his home in the *Old Town*. The crumbling edifices of the University and the College of Physicians contrasted with William Adam's immaculate Royal Infirmary. Lord Provost Drummond planned to build a better Edinburgh. In 1775, Cullen, as President of the College, laid the foundation stone of one of the first public buildings in the *New Town* – the Physicians' Hall in George Street. The concluding sections, *Biography and remembrances*, focus on the two volume biography of Cullen by John Thomson and on the memorabilia displayed in the exhibition.

Boyhood in Lanarkshire

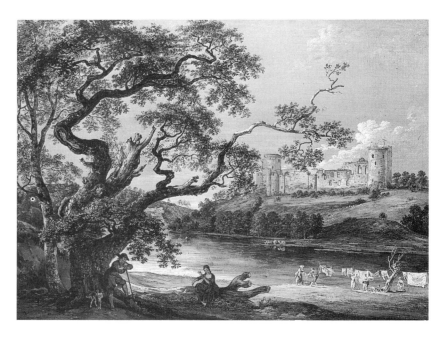

1. **Bothwell Castle**   *Fig. 1*
Watercolour by Paul Sandby
Colour photograph: National Gallery of Scotland

Many of Cullen's happiest childhood memories were of the Clyde
Valley where his family had a small estate near Bothwell Castle.

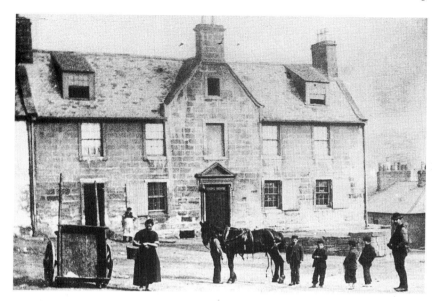

2. **Hamilton Grammar School**   *Fig. 2*
Photograph: Hamilton District Museum

Cullen received his school education in this building more than
150 years before this photograph was taken. It was erected, in
1711, by Anne, Duchess of Hamilton. Her grandson, the 5th Duke
of Hamilton, attended as a pupil for five years before going to
Eton.

3. **General View of Hamilton** 1825
Watercolour by I. Clark
Colour photograph: Hamilton District Museum

Cullen spent most of his school days in Hamilton where his father
was a lawyer and factor to the Duke of Hamilton.

General practice in Hamilton

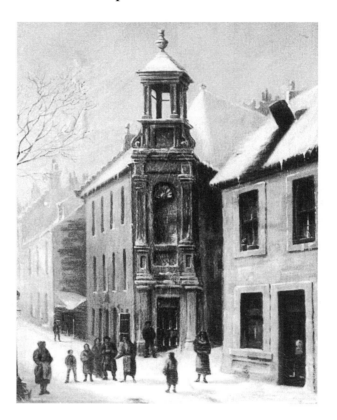

4. **Duchess Anne's Almshouse and William Cullen's** *Fig. 3*
House in Hamilton
Oil painting attributed to Sam Bough
Colour photograph: Hamilton District Museum

The almshouse is the building surmounted by a small belfry and
Cullen's house is the thatched building on the right.

5. **James, 5th Duke of Hamilton** (1703–43)

Oil painting by William Aikman
Collection at Lennoxlove
Colour photograph: Scottish National Portrait Gallery

Cullen was the ordinary medical attendant to the Duke and his family. He was also responsible for some veterinary duties on the Hamilton estates. The Duke persuaded Cullen to stay on in Hamilton by promising to equip a chemical laboratory for him and to make him superintendent of the Palace botanic gardens. The promise was not fulfilled because of the Duke's premature death.

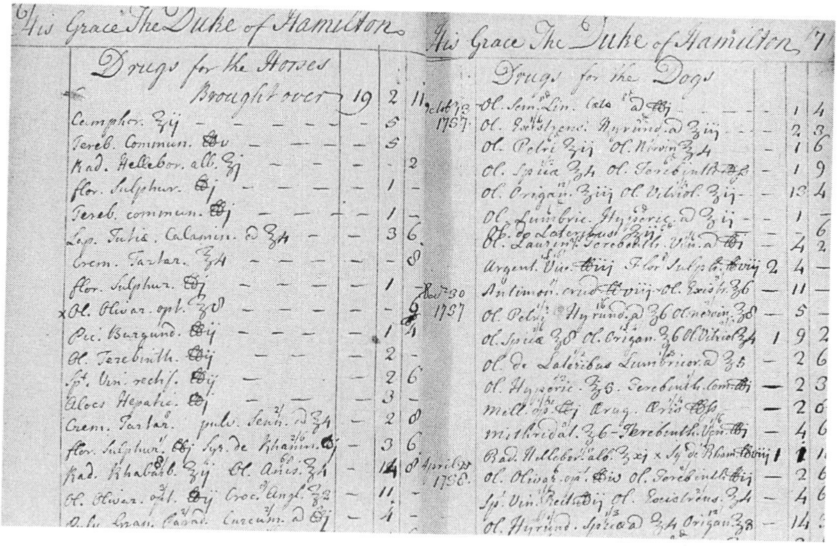

6. **'Account Book**, containing the record of medicines and medicinal preparations furnished by Dr William Cullen at Hamilton, 1737–41' Royal College of Physicians of Edinburgh MS Cullen 34

Fig. 4

The entries in the ledger include veterinary preparations for the Duke of Hamilton's dogs and horses.

Lads o' pairts

William Cullen was one of four Lanarkshire boys, born within
thirty years and thirty miles of each other, who later achieved
international fame in medicine. Cullen's three contemporaries
were:
William Smellie (Lanark). The master of British midwifery
William Hunter (East Kilbride). Celebrated anatomist and
obstetrician
John Hunter (East Kilbride). The founder of surgical science.

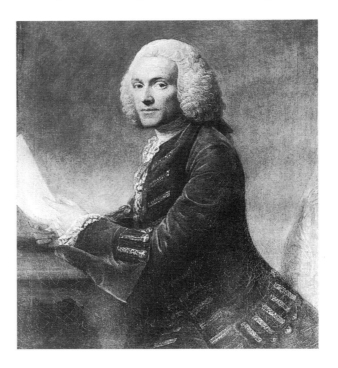

7. **William Hunter** (1718–83)   *Fig. 5*
Anatomist and obstetrician
Oil painting by Allan Ramsay
Colour photograph: Hunterian Art Gallery, University of Glasgow

William Hunter was Cullen's surgeon apothecary apprentice in
Hamilton, where he lived in his master's house. Hunter later
described this period as the three happiest years of his life.

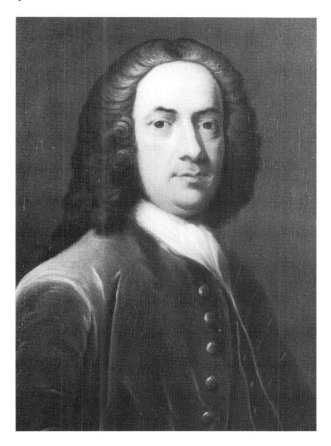

8. **William Smellie** (1697–1763)   *Fig. 6*
Obstetrician
Oil painting; self-portrait
Colour photograph: Royal College of Surgeons
of Edinburgh

A Lanarkshire friend of Cullen who became one of Britain's leading obstetricians. Despite great opposition, from midwives and prudes, he succeeded in bringing obstetrics within the orbit of medicine. Shortly after setting up practice in London, William Hunter arrived with a letter of introduction from Cullen. Hunter lived with Smellie and his wife during his first year in London.

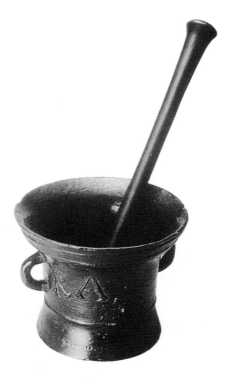

9. **Pestle and Mortar**   *Fig. 7*
Royal College of Physicians of Edinburgh

In his early career, as a surgeon apothecary, Cullen dispensed his own drugs. Traditionally, this pestle and mortar belonged to him.

University of Glasgow

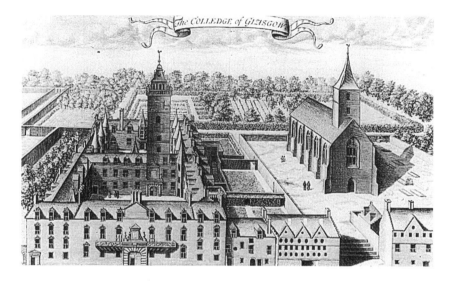

10. **Glasgow University**   *Fig. 8*
J. Slezer *Theatrum Scotiae*, London, 1693
Photograph: Medical Illustration, University of Edinburgh

Cullen was the first holder of the lectureship in chemistry, which
Glasgow University instituted in 1747. When he became professor
of medicine in 1751, Cullen changed the nature of the appointment
from a titular sinecure to a teaching post. He was one of the
principal founders of the Glasgow Medical School.

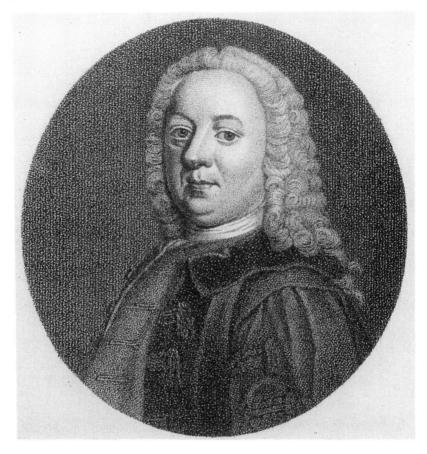

11. **Robert Simson** (1687–1768)   *Fig. 9*
Mathematician
Engraving by A. Baillie after W. Denune
Photograph: Medical Illustration, University of Edinburgh

Simson was one of the most learned and engaging professors in Glasgow. His studies in geometry helped to make this subject the core of Scottish mathematics during the eighteenth and early nineteenth centuries. He influenced William Cullen and Adam Smith when they were his students and both retained a life-long interest in mathematics. They later enjoyed his support as young professors.

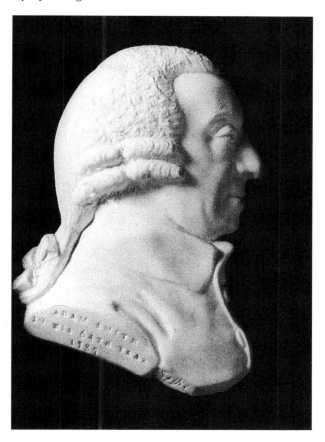

12. **Adam Smith** (1723–90) *Fig. 10*
Philosopher and economist
Paste medallion by James Tassie
Colour photograph: Scottish National Portrait Gallery

In 1751, Adam Smith and William Cullen gained their first
university chairs in Glasgow, within a few days of each other.
Smith was appointed to the chair of logic and later became
professor of moral philosophy. They became lifelong friends.

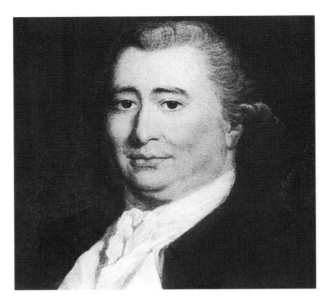

13. **David Hume** (1711–76)   *Fig. 11*
Philosopher and historian
Oil painting by Lady Abercromby
Colour photograph: Edinburgh University

When David Hume was a candidate for the chair of logic in Glasgow, in 1752, he received strong support from William Cullen. Adam Smith had some reservations which he expressed to Cullen:

'I should prefer David Hume to any man for a colleague; but I am afraid the public would not be of my opinion; and the interest of the society will oblige us to have some regard to the opinion of the public.'

Hume was unsuccessful in his application but, within a few days he was appointed Keeper of the Advocates' Library in Edinburgh.

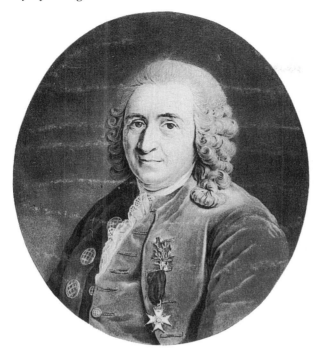

14. **Carl Linnaeus** (1707–78)   *Fig. 12*
Botanist and physician
Lithograph by P.M. Alix after A. Roslin
Thomson Walker Collection,
TW2, L1
Photograph: Edinburgh University Library

The botany lectures which Cullen gave in Glasgow between 1747 and 1750 were delivered in Latin. He used the newly introduced classification of Linnaeus. Cullen later admitted that when he first read Linnaeus' botanical system the language in which it was expressed appeared to him 'a piece of the most uncouth jargon and minute pedantry' that he had ever seen; but with the passage of time it became as familiar to him as his mother-tongue.

Chemistry

William Cullen was an influential figure in the development of chemistry. He was one of the first to succeed in establishing the subject as a science in its own right, because of its importance to industry and agriculture. His critical outlook and innovative methods of instruction contributed to his reputation as a teacher. In Edinburgh the number of students attending his chemistry course rose from 17 in the first year to 59 in the second and so on until he had a class of 145.

15. **John Locke** *An essay concerning human understanding*
2 vols in 4, 11th edition, London, 1835: title page and author's portrait
Photograph: Edinburgh University Library

At the beginning of his course in chemistry it was Cullen's custom to advise his students to read Locke's *Essay*:

'I shall now proceed to give some advice with regard to your Conduct in Theoretical enquiries . . . But to enable you to follow me, and to make any advances yourselves in Chemical philosophy, much preparatory knowledge is necessary. Logic is a very necessary part of the introductory learning; by logic I mean the analysis of the human mind, such as may be found in Mr Locke's excellent treatise of the understanding. This is not only necessary in Chemistry, but also in every Science where there is danger of error.' (Royal College of Physicians of Edinburgh Cullen MS 10, vol. 1, 26–27.)

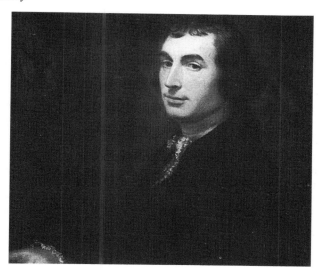

16. **Joseph Black** (1728–99)   *Fig. 13*
Chemist and physician
Oil painting by David Martin
Colour photograph: University of Edinburgh

Black studied medicine in Glasgow and Edinburgh. His interest in chemistry was aroused in Glasgow by Cullen. Of this period he wrote:

'Dr Cullen about this time began also to give lectures on Chemistry which had never before been taught in the University of Glasgow and finding that I might be useful to him in that undertaking employed me as his assistant in the laboratory and treated me with the same confidence and friendship and direction in my studies, as if I had been one of his children.' (Edinburgh University Library MS Dc.2.76[8])

17. **Joseph Black** *De Humore Acido a Cibis Orto, et Magnesia Alba*
M.D. thesis, Edinburgh University, 1754: title page
Photograph: Edinburgh University Library

In this thesis, dedicated to William Cullen, Joseph Black records his discovery of 'fixed air' or carbon dioxide. He was the first person to use a balance in a planned set of experiments and thus laid the foundations of modern quantitative chemistry.

18. **William Cullen** 'Of the cold produced by
evaporating fluids and of some other means of producing cold'.
Essays and Observations, Physical and Literary
[Edinburgh Philosophical Society] 1756; 2:145–56

The observations made by Cullen on evaporative cooling played a
part in turning Joseph Black's thoughts in the direction which led
to his discovery of latent and specific heat.

19. **Andrew Plummer** (1698–1756)
Chemist and physician
Oil painting by John Alexander
Colour photograph: Miss A. Scott-Plummer

Plummer studied medicine and chemistry under Boerhaave, in
Leiden. He was appointed professor of chemistry and medicine in
Edinburgh when the Faculty of Medicine was founded in 1726.
After Plummer became incapacitated by illness, in late 1755,
Cullen was appointed professor of chemistry in association with
Plummer. When he died, the following year, Cullen became the
sole occupant of the chair of chemistry.

20. **A Brain Chain: Teacher and Student from Cullen to Graham**

William Cullen (1710–90) Promoted chemistry as a scientific
discipline

Joseph Black (1728–99) Discovered carbon dioxide and latent
heat. Developed the concept of specific heat.

Daniel Rutherford (1749–1819)
Discovered nitrogen

Thomas Thomson (1773–1852) Performed pioneer studies in heat
conduction, densitometry and mineralogy

Thomas Graham (1805–69) Made fundamental observations in
the diffusion of gases (Graham's Law), colloids,
crystalloids and dialysis

Bleaching of linen

During the 18th century, linen manufacture in Scotland developed from a small backward craft into a major British industry. Aid to improve the manufacturing process came from the Board of Trustees for Fisheries and Manufactures. The Board recognised that there was a particular need to improve the methods used to bleach linen and requested Francis Home, William Cullen and others to apply their chemical expertise to this problem.

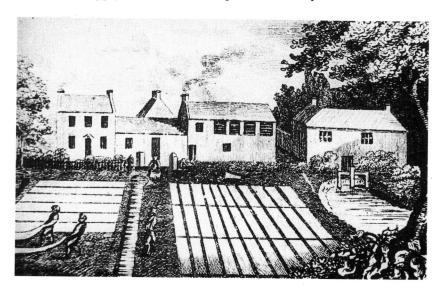

21. **Falkirk Bleach-Fields**   *Fig. 14*
Drawing
Photograph: Falkirk Museums

Cullen experienced difficulty in explaining the bleaching produced by laying cloth out in sunlight.

22. **Francis Home** *Experiments on bleaching*
Edinburgh, 1756

Reference is made to Cullen's work on bleaching. The results of
Home's experiments led to the replacement of sour milk by dilute
sulphuric acid in bleaching, and shortened the process by several
days. Cullen was less successful than Home in his experiments,
which were designed to find a cheaper and more reliable source of
alkali, for bleaching, than wood ashes, which were imported from
Sweden and Russia. The problem was not fully solved until after
Cullen's death when sodium hypochlorite was introduced.

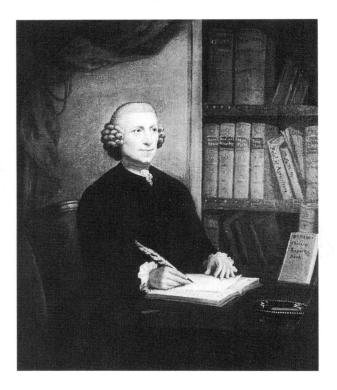

23. **Francis Home** (1719–1813)   *Fig. 15*
Professor of materia medica, Edinburgh University
Oil painting attributed to David Allan
Colour photograph: University of Edinburgh

Francis Home made several notable contributions to medicine,
agriculture and applied chemistry.

Agriculture

Cullen applied his knowledge of chemistry and botany to agricultural improvement. He witnessed practical results on the farm of Parkhead, in Lanarkshire, which he managed for his brother; and later, on his own farm, at Ormiston Hill in Midlothian. His influence on agricultural progress is assessed by C.W.J. Withers, 'William Cullen's agricultural lectures and writings and the development of agricultural science in eighteenth century Scotland', *Ag. Hist. Rev.* 1989; 37, pt 11: 144–56.

24. **William Cullen** 'The substance of nine lectures on vegetation and agriculture, delivered to a private audience in the year 1768'. In: *Additional appendix to . . . the proposed general report from the Board of Agriculture on the subject of manures* London, 1796

In these lectures, published in abridged form posthumously, Cullen concentrates particularly on the chemical and physical means of improving soil fertility. At the conclusion of the lecture series he remarks: '. . . if, after trial, any of you shall find the above theory in any respect contrary to practice, it will do me a singular pleasure to be acquainted with it, that I may correct my errors. Truth, and the advancement of an art so useful to mankind, is my sole object; and to attain this I hope, I shall be ever ready to sacrifice any theory, however dear it may formerly have been held.'

25. **Andrew Coventry MD** (1764–1832)
Professor of agriculture, Edinburgh University,
Paste medallion by James Tassie
Photograph: Scottish National Portrait Gallery

Andrew Coventry was appointed to the first chair of agriculture in Britain, founded in Edinburgh in 1790 by Sir William Pulteney. During his medical studies Coventry came under the influence of three professors who contributed to agricultural improvement: Francis Home (materia medica), William Cullen (medicine) and John Hope (botany).

Cullen's patrons

In eighteenth century Scotland appointments to university chairs were strongly influenced by the political patronage system, which often acted on the advice of notable professional men. Through common interests in chemistry, agriculture and industrial improvement, Cullen gained the patronage of the Duke of Argyll and the support of Lord Kames.

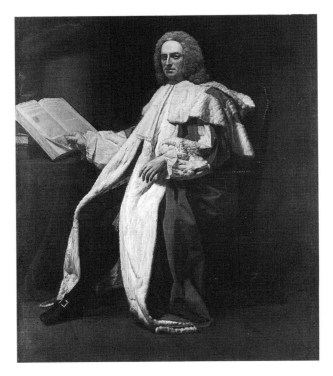

26. **Archibald Campbell, 3rd Duke of Argyll** (1682–1761) *Fig. 16*
Lawyer and politician
Oil painting by Allan Ramsay
Colour photograph: Glasgow Art Gallery and Museum

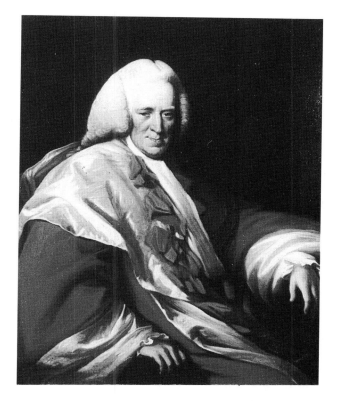

27. Henry Home, Lord Kames (1696–1782) *Fig. 17*
Judge, agriculturalist and philosopher
Oil painting by David Martin
Colour photograph: Scottish National Portrait Gallery

Kames published influential work on the law, literary criticism and agriculture. He encouraged Cullen to move to Edinburgh.

The Duke of Argyll, formerly Lord Ilay, was successful in influencing the Government in the interests of Scotland. He patronised men who aided his scientific pursuits, and was equally at ease with high and low, a gift which brought him the admiration of those who served him, and the exasperation of his opponents. Against considerable local opposition, he played a decisive role in securing Cullen's appointment to the chair of chemistry in Edinburgh.

28. **Letter From Henry Home (Lord Kames)**
to Lord Milton seeking his support for Cullen's
appointment to the chair of chemistry in Edinburgh
National Library of Scotland MS 16692, f.101
Colour laser photocopy: Trustees of the National
Library of Scotland

Kames 6 Sep: 1755

My Lord

When any thing occurs for the good of the Publick, I naturally cast
my eyes upon your Lordship, as the fittest Person in Scotland for
carrying on every work of this kind – Dr Plummer is dead and the
properest man in Great Britain to succeed to the Profession of
Chymistry is Dr Cullen – He will infallibly raise the reputation of
that College which at present is sunk very low; and this in all
probability will draw strangers in great abundance to study at
Edinburgh. I am I confess the more solicitous about this matter
that I know Cullen to be a fast adherent to the Duke of Argyll, and
that his Grace has a good opinion of him. I know at the same time
that the Doctor is so well esteemed in Edinburgh, that it will
require no more to make the Point effectual, than your Lordships
declaring for him.

I am with the greatest respect
  Your Lordships
    devoted servant
      Henry Home

Lord Milton was the Duke of Argyll's principal agent in Scotland.
This letter was prompted by a report of the death of Dr Plummer,
professor of chemistry in the University of Edinburgh, which was
later found to be incorrect. Plummer had a stroke and survived for
a year.

Infirmary teaching

The Edinburgh Medical School was founded in 1726 and was the first English-speaking school to provide a full range of medical training. Within fifty years it had gained the reputation of being the best medical school in Europe. A major factor in its early success was the clinical teaching in its large voluntary hospital – Edinburgh Royal Infirmary.

The Hospital was designed by William Adam to accommodate 228 patients. The building was sited close to the university and was constructed in stages, the first patients being admitted in 1741. In 1879 the Adam Infirmary was replaced by the present Royal Infirmary building at Lauriston Place.

During the first half of his Edinburgh career, Cullen looked after patients in the Infirmary and was involved in clinical teaching. On his arrival from Glasgow he was granted permission to use one of the Infirmary's vaulted kitchens for experiments connected with the teaching of chemistry, but later obtained more appropriate laboratory accommodation outwith the hospital.

29. **Royal Infirmary of Edinburgh in the Eighteenth Century**
Model (1:50 scale) by David Montgomery, 1987
Royal Infirmary of Edinburgh

Architect: William Adam (1689–1748)
Built: 1738–48. Demolished: 1884.

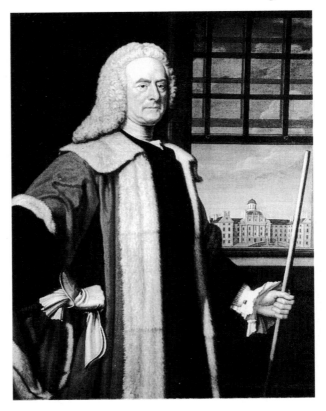

30. **George Drummond** (1687–1766)   *Fig. 18*
Financier and politician
Oil painting by John Alexander
Colour photograph: Royal Infirmary of Edinburgh

Drummond was a man of vision and Edinburgh's greatest Lord
Provost. He raised funds to build the Royal Infirmary (seen
through the window in this picture) and was the driving force
behind the creation of the New Town. As civic head he presided
over the expansion of the Medical School. During this period, the
University was under the management of the Town Council.
Cullen appreciated Drummond's advice on difficulties which he
experienced in establishing his career in Edinburgh.

Lectures in clinical medicine

The teaching of clinical medicine attracted increasing numbers of students after the introduction, in 1757, of a conjoint course of lectures in which the professor of medicine, John Rutherford, was joined by three professorial colleagues:
Alexander Monro *primus*
Robert Whytt
William Cullen

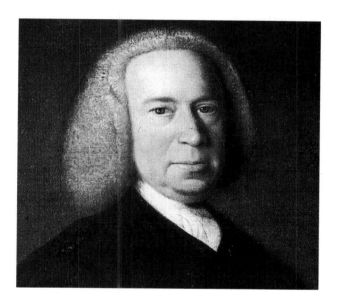

31. **John Rutherford** (1695–1779)   *Fig. 19*
Physician
Oil painting by William Millar
Colour photograph: Mrs P.M. Maxwell-Scott

Rutherford was professor of the practice of physic and a founder member of the Faculty of Medicine. A fervent disciple of Boerhaave he adopted his system of teaching and was the first in Edinburgh to deliver lectures in clinical medicine at the Infirmary. He was the maternal grandfather of Sir Walter Scott and the father of Daniel Rutherford who discovered nitrogen.

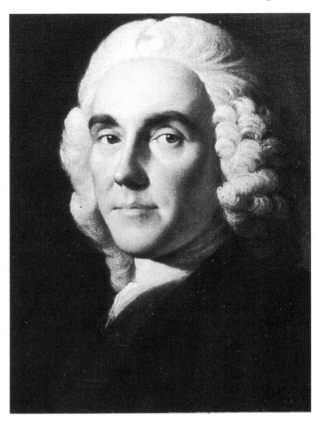

32 **Alexander Monro** *primus* (1697–1767)   *Fig. 20*
Anatomist, surgeon and physician
Oil painting by Allan Ramsay
Colour photograph: private owner of portrait

Dr Alexander Monro *primus* is 'not content with barely teaching anatomy he launches out into all the branches of physick where all his remarks are new and useful . . . he is not only a skilful physician but an able orator and delivers things in their nature abstruse in so easy a manner that the most unlearn'd may, must understand him' – Oliver Goldsmith (K.C. Balderstone *Collected letters of Oliver Goldsmith*, Cambridge, 1928:6).

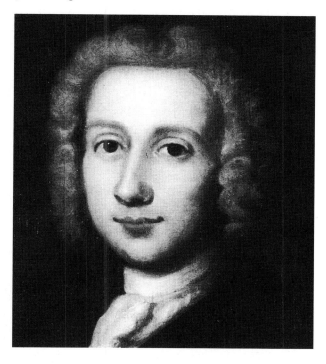

33. **Robert Whytt** (1714–66)   *Fig. 21*
Physiologist and physician
Oil painting by an unknown artist after the school of Bellucci
Colour photograph: Royal College of Physicians of Edinburgh

Professor of the institutes of medicine and the practice of
medicine, Whytt contributed materially to the rise of Edinburgh as
an international medical centre, because of his original work in
neurology. He performed fundamental experiments on reflex
action and provided early accurate descriptions of several diseases
of the brain.

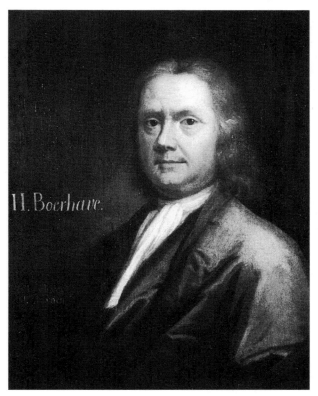

34. **Herman Boerhaave** (1668–1738)   *Fig. 22*
Professor of medicine, chemistry and botany in
the University of Leiden
Oil painting by an unknown artist
Colour photograph: Royal College of Physicians of London

This great teacher was the central figure of European medicine in
the first half of the 18th century and he was highly influential in the
development of the Edinburgh Medical School. He taught
medicine as a practical skill, not as a theoretical subject. Most of
the first generation of professors in the Edinburgh Faculty were
former students of Boerhaave and taught his system of medicine.

35. Edinburgh's Reaction to Cullen's Modification of the Boerhaavian System

Extract from an introductory lecture delivered by William Cullen to his Edinburgh medical students in the 1783–84 course on the practice of physic (John Thomson *An account of the life, lectures and writings of William Cullen MD*, 2 vols, Edinburgh, 1859; 1:118–119)

'Soon after I came here, I was engaged to give clinical, that is practical, lectures; and in these I ventured to give my own opinion of the nature and cure of diseases, different in several respects from that of the Boerhaavians. This soon produced an outcry against me . . . This went so far, that my friend and patron, the late George Drummond, whose venerable bust you see in the hall of the Infirmary, came to me, requesting seriously that I would avoid differing from Dr Boerhaave, as he found my conduct in that respect was likely to hurt myself and the University also. I promised to be cautious; . . . as I truly esteem Dr Boerhaave as a philosopher, a physician, and the author of a system more perfect than any thing that had gone before, and as perfect as the state of science in this time would permit of . . . I was, however, no violent reformer; and, by degrees only, I ventured to point out the imperfections, and even the errors, of Dr Boerhaave's system . . .'

36. *Fidem Non Derogat Error*

Inscription on a students' class card issued for
Cullen's course on the practice of medicine,
1775.
Photograph: Edinburgh University Library

This maxim was exemplified by Cullen in a clinical lecture: 'it is not improperly said that the earth hides the faults of the physician. If every patient that dies were opened, as ours has been, it would but too often discover the frivolity of our conjectures and practice . . . with regard to the present case, I might go back to consider the symptoms, and from them endeavour to account for my own ignorance; but I choose rather to acknowledge my mistakes, and to consider the case on the footing which we have now learned from dissection.' (Thomson, see above, 1: 108–09)

University teaching

Cullen was one of the greatest medical teachers of his age. Among the many qualities admired by his students were his clarity of thought and expression, his vivacity, his candour and his excellence in communicating ideas and stimulating enthusiasm for self learning. Cullen's lectures were delivered with only brief reference to notes; he considered that lectures given in language fit to print were too stiff and formal.

37. **William Cullen** *Lectures on chymistry*
1763–64, vol. 1
Manuscript notes
The Honourable Lord Cullen

Cullen's method of representing the course of certain chemical reactions by the use of arrows was an important step in the teaching of chemistry in the eighteenth century. It is now appreciated that some of the contributions to the theory of affinity previously credited to the Swedish chemist, Torbern Bergman (e.g. the concept of double elective attraction and the effect of heat on affinities), are based on ideas developed by William Cullen and Joseph Black in their lectures in Edinburgh.

38. **William Cullen** *Lectures on the institutions of medicine*
5 vols, 1770
Royal College of Physicians of Edinburgh, Cullen MS 18

These notes were taken by a student and may have been transcribed in a fair hand by a 'professional' copyist. They consist of lectures on Physiology (vols. 1–3), Pathology (vol. 4) and Therapeutics (vol. 5). In many ways these verbatim accounts provide a better understanding of Cullen's thinking and teaching than his published work.

39. **William Cullen** *Lectures on physiology*
2 vols, *c.*1766
Royal College of Physicians of Edinburgh, Cullen MS 16

These are bound copies of Cullen's own notes, folded in typical fashion which he is seen holding in the portrait by Cochrane (see frontispiece).

40. **William Cullen** *Lectures on pathology*
2 vols, *c.*1766
Royal College of Physicians of Edinburgh, Cullen MS 28

In his own hand Cullen outlines his principles of general pathology with a few references to morbid anatomical changes. Factors involved in the causation of disease and the production of symptoms are considered in detail.

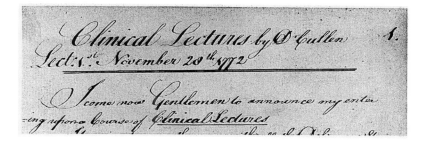

41 **William Cullen** *Clinical lectures* *Fig. 23*
4 vols, 1772–73
Royal College of Physicians of Edinburgh, Cullen MS 4; 1: title on p.1

This is one of the most detailed sets of notes taken from Cullen's lectures on clinical medicine. Cullen's skill as a teacher is revealed in his discussion of a wide range of diseases.

Bibliophile and author

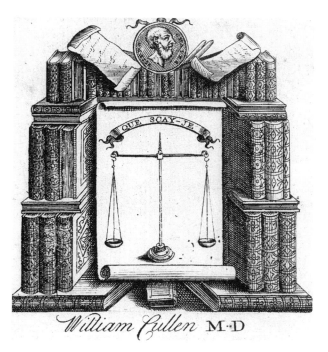

42. Book Plate of William Cullen   *Fig. 24*
Royal College of Physicians of Edinburgh

This plate is affixed to the inside board of *Traité du mouvement et de la mesure des eaux coulantes et jaillisantes* . . . by Pierre Varignon, Paris, 1725. The work was bought for one shilling by the College at the sale of Dr Cullen's books.

It would seem that Cullen appreciated the sceptical ideas associated with Montaigne's motto 'What do I know?' inscribed over a pair of scales in balance.

43. *[Sale] Catalogue of [Dr Cullen's]*
Medical Books, [1792]
Royal College of Physicians of Edinburgh

Cullen's scholarship owed much to his breadth and depth of
reading in the arts, science and medicine. During his lifetime he
built up a fine private library which he made freely available to
his students and friends. Most of the books which he wrote on
medical subjects ran through a number of editions and were
translated into several languages. The greater part of Dr Cullen's
library was sold after his death. The sale catalogue lists 3,765 items
and includes a significant number of non-medical works. Most of
the books were published in the seventeenth and eighteenth
centuries and many are written in Latin, French and other
European languages.

44. **William Cullen** *Physiologie*
French translation by E.F.M. Bosquillon, Paris, 1785
Royal College of Physicians of Edinburgh

This book is a translation of the third edition of Cullen's
Institutions of medicine, part I, physiology, which was also
published in 1785. The work was first published in 1772 for the
benefit of Cullen's students. On his appointment to the Edinburgh
chair of medicine, in 1773, he ceased giving lectures on the
institutes of medicine and published no further work under this
title.

45. **William Cullen** *Synopsis Nosologiae Methodicae*
2nd edition, Edinburgh, 1772
Royal College of Physicians of Edinburgh

Cullen's book on disease classifications, including his own nosology,
was first published in Latin in 1769 for the use of his students. He
used a revised version of his nosology, published in the second
edition of *Synopsis Nosologiae Methodicae*, to structure his *First
Lines of the Practice of Physic* (1777–84). When used together
these two works provide a valuable source of information on the
eighteenth century definitions and nomenclature of symptoms and
disease.

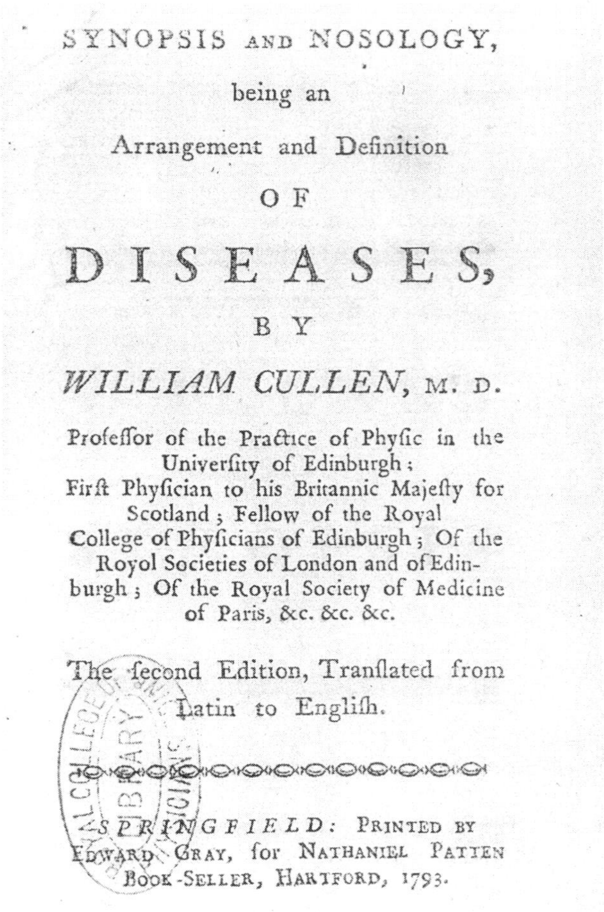

SYNOPSIS AND NOSOLOGY,

being an

Arrangement and Definition

O F

D I S E A S E S,

B Y

WILLIAM CULLEN, M. D.

Profeffor of the Practice of Phyfic in the
Univerfity of Edinburgh;
Firft Phyfician to his Britannic Majefty for
Scotland; Fellow of the Royal
College of Phyficians of Edinburgh; Of the
Royol Societies of London and of Edin-
burgh; Of the Royal Society of Medicine
of Paris, &c. &c. &c.

The fecond Edition, Tranflated from
Latin to Englifh.

S P R I N G F I E L D: PRINTED BY
EDWARD GRAY, for NATHANIEL PATTEN
BOOK-SELLER, HARTFORD, 1793.

46. William Cullen *Synopsis and nosology,*   *Fig. 25*
being an arrangement and definition of diseases
Translation from Latin to English,
Springfield, Connecticut, 1793.
Royal College of Physicians of Edinburgh

On display, next to the above, were the English translation
published in Edinburgh in 1815 and the London Latin edition of
1823 which also includes an English translation.

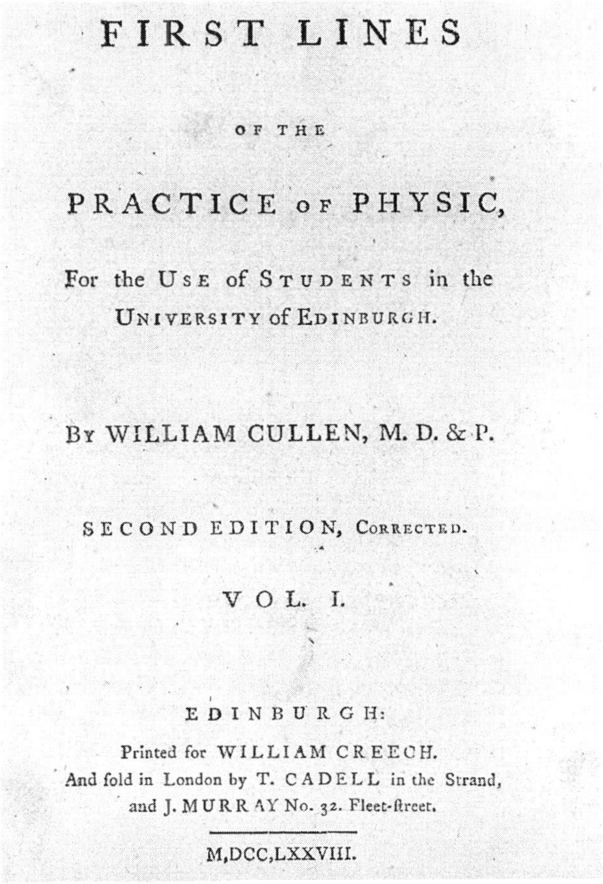

FIRST LINES

OF THE

PRACTICE OF PHYSIC,

For the USE of STUDENTS in the
UNIVERSITY of EDINBURGH.

By WILLIAM CULLEN, M. D. & P.

SECOND EDITION, CORRECTED.

VOL. I.

EDINBURGH:

Printed for WILLIAM CREECH.
And fold in London by T. CADELL in the Strand,
and J. MURRAY No. 32. Fleet-ftreet.

M,DCC,LXXVIII.

47. **William Cullen** *First lines of the practice of physic*   *Fig. 26*
4 vols in 6, 2nd edition, Edinburgh, 1778–84
Royal College of Physicians of Edinburgh.

This work was translated into French, German, Italian and Latin
and retained its position as a leading text book on the practice of
medicine for more than fifty years. The set of volumes displayed
belonged to the author and show his annotations. As with many
medical works, the process of expansion and revision went on side
by side with consequent confusion in the description of editions.
The fourth volume first appeared in 1784 and is entitled 'Second
edition'.

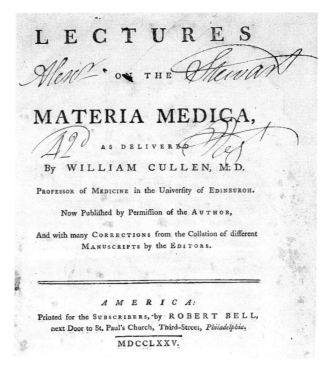

48. William Cullen *Lectures on the materia medica*   *Fig. 27*
Philadelphia, 1775
Royal College of Physicians of Edinburgh

In 1772 a pirated edition of Cullen's lectures on the materia medica, which he had given eleven years previously, was published in London. Cullen took out an injunction to prevent the sale of further copies. He later agreed to a reissue of the work, with a supplement to correct the many errors; this was published in London in 1773, and in Philadelphia two years later (see pp. 92–93).

49. **William Cullen** *A treatise of the materia medica*
Author's proof copy, 2 vols in 1, Edinburgh, *c.*1788
Royal College of Physicians of Edinburgh

Towards the end of his life, Cullen devoted much time to this work, extensively revising his lectures on the materia medica which had been previously published and adding a large amount of new material. The amendments in this proof copy are in the hand of Cullen and of his last amanuensis, Mr. Paul.

50. **William Cullen** *A treatise of the materia medica*
2 vols, Edinburgh, 1789
Royal College of Physicians of Edinburgh

This treatise was widely used throughout Europe and North America and was translated into German and French. It remained a standard work for about forty years.

Cullen was among the first to attempt the classification of medicines according to their physiological action and their effects as ascertained by observation and clinical experiments. The classification met with limited success because physiology and pharmacology were not sufficiently advanced to allow him to base it on reliable scientific information.

Cullen's influence on American medicine

During the eighteenth century the Edinburgh Medical School became the most influential European school in the development of American medicine as described fully by Dr O'Donnell on pp. 234–46. In the second half of the century 117 Americans gained their medical degree at Edinburgh and a large number attended medical courses without graduating.

Among the Edinburgh medical teachers it was William Cullen who, almost without exception, won the admiration and affection of the Americans.

'. . . the great unrivalled Dr Cullen'   Benjamin Rush

'. . . that shining oracle of physic'   Thomas Parke

Foundation of the Medical School of the College of Philadelphia – the first medical school in North America

The school was founded in 1765 by John Morgan who worked on his plans while abroad and discussed them with William Cullen, John Fothergill and William Hunter. Morgan was of the firm opinion that a medical school should not be a private undertaking but an integral part of a college or university. He used Edinburgh as his example which demonstrated the fruitful results of 'united efforts of men learned in their professions' who not only brought world-wide fame to their city and their university, but also advanced science.

The first professors of the Faculty were all Edinburgh-trained and former pupils of William Cullen: John Morgan, William Shippen, Benjamin Rush and Adam Kuhn.

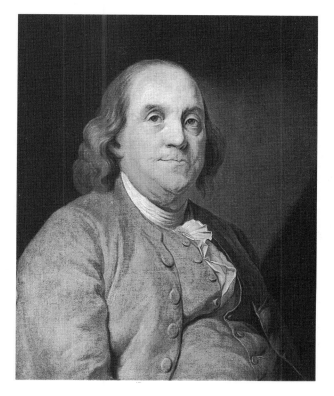

51. **Benjamin Franklin** (1706–90)   *Fig. 28*
Scientist and statesman
Oil painting after Joseph Siffred Duplessis
Colour photograph: National Portrait Gallery, London

Franklin acted as adviser and sponsor to a whole generation of Americans abroad. He introduced students by personal letters to Cullen and to Cullen's friends, John Fothergill and William Hunter in London. Franklin had no hesitation in directing his protégés to Edinburgh for medicine despite this autobiographical remark:

'A disputatious turn, by the way, is apt to become a very bad habit, making people often very disagreeable in company . . . Persons of good sense, I have since observed, seldom fall into it, except lawyers, University men and men of allsorts that have been bred at Edinburgh.'

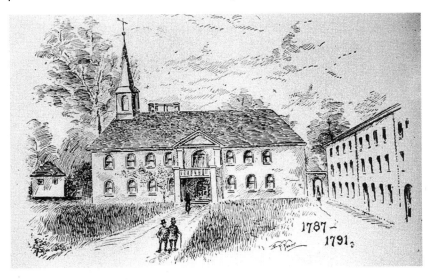

52. The College of Philadelphia   *Fig. 29*
Drawing by E.F. Faber
Photograph: College of Physicians of Philadelphia

The origin of the College of Philadelphia dates from 1740 with the creation of a free school trust which led to the development of an academy. A new charter in 1755 changed the name to the College of Philadelphia and permitted the institution to broaden its curriculum and award academic degrees. The first provost of the College was the Reverend William Smith from Aberdeenshire who planned the curriculum along lines familiar to the Scottish university tradition. Among the first arts graduates was John Morgan who later founded the College's medical school. In 1791 the College became the University of Pennsylvania.

When the College of Physicians of Philadelphia was founded in 1787 it held its meetings, until 1791, in rooms rented from the College of Philadelphia.

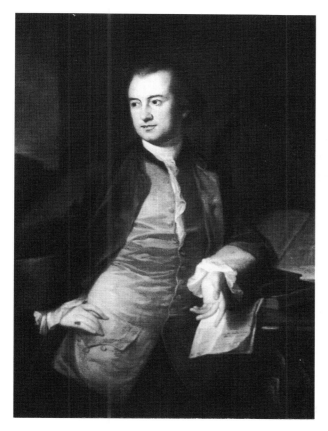

53. John Morgan (1753–89)   *Fig. 30*
Professor of the theory and practice of physic
Oil painting by Vincent Desiderio after the original by Angelica
Kauffmann
Colour photograph: Royal College of Physicians of Edinburgh

The first medical professor in British North America and the
'father of American medicine'. In recommending Morgan as a
student to Cullen, Benjamin Franklin said of him: 'Mr Morgan
. . . is a young gentleman of Philadelphia, whom I have long
known and greatly esteem; and as I interest myself in what relates
to him, I cannot but wish him the advantage of your conversation
and instructions. I wish it also for the sake of my country, where he
is to reside, and where I am persuaded he will be not a little
useful.' (J. Thomson, *An Account of the life, lectures and writings
of William Cullen MD*, 2 vols, Edinburgh, 1859; 1:140.)

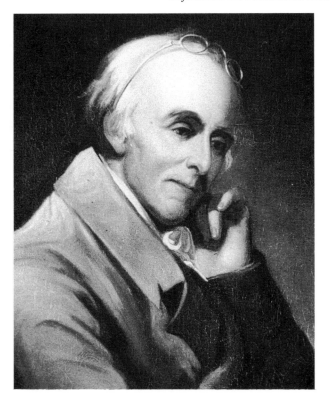

54. **Benjamin Rush** (1745–1813)   *Fig. 31*
Professor of chemistry and medicine
Oil painting by Thomas Sully
Colour photograph: Independence National
Historical Park Collection, Philadelphia

Rush later became professor of the theory and practice of
medicine in the College of Philadelphia and professor of the
institutes of medicine in the University of Pennsylvania. He was
the only medical signatory of the Declaration of Independence. A
passionate reformer and tireless writer, Rush promoted many
worthy causes – the abolition of slavery, education, prison reform,
medical care for the poor and humane treatment of the insane.

During the American War of Independence Rush had Cullen's
First lines of the practice of physic published in Philadelphia: 'Sir,
you see you have had a hand in the Revolution by contributing
indirectly to save the lives of officers and soldiers of the American
Army'.

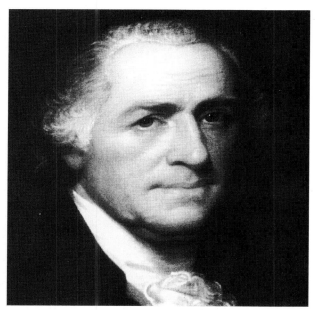

55. **William Shippen,** *Jun.* (1736–1808)   *Fig. 32*
Professor of anatomy and surgery
Oil painting by Gilbert Stuart
Photograph: College of Physicians of Philadelphia

Before coming to Edinburgh, where he graduated M.D. in 1761, William Shippen had obtained an arts degree and served a medical apprenticeship in America. He had also acquired a sound practical training in anatomy from John and William Hunter, in London. For Shippen, Edinburgh's attraction was the teaching of William Cullen and Alexander Monro *secundus*. He appreciated Cullen's hospitality and many years later reminded him that he was the pupil who 'was as fond of a Solan Goose as you were'.

Shippen returned to Philadelphia before the medical school was founded and gave private lectures in anatomy and in midwifery. Although he encountered opposition from midwives who resented his encroachment on their field, this was shortlived because he encouraged them to attend his lectures and seek his clinical assistance in difficult cases. Shippen was the first doctor in America to give courses of systematic instruction on obstetrics and he became professor of midwifery some years after his appointment to the chair of anatomy and surgery. Rush described Shippen's teaching as 'eloquent, pleasing and luminous'.

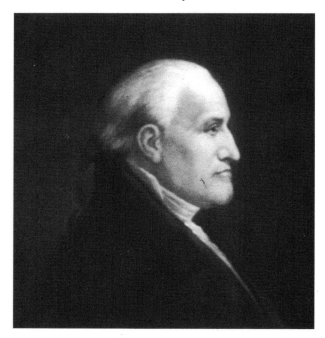

56. **Adam Kuhn** (1741–1817)   *Fig. 33*
Professor of botany and materia medica
Oil painting by Louis Hasselbusch
Photograph: College of Physicians of Philadelphia

Kuhn studied botany under Carl Linnaeus at Uppsala before
pursuing his undergraduate medical training in Edinburgh.

57. *A Tribute presented by the City of*
Philadelphia to the Royal College of Physicians
of Edinburgh upon the occasion of its
Tercentenary. September 6, 1981.
Illuminated address

This Address bears the signature of William Green, Mayor of the
City of Philadelphia. It pays tribute to Edinburgh's medical
organisations for training the young Americans who later played a
major role in establishing the first medical school in North
America and the College of Physicians in Philadelphia.

Cullen was their mentor

58. **Joseph Black** (1728–99)
Chemist and physician
Oil painting by Sir Henry Raeburn
Colour photograph: Hunterian Art Gallery,
University of Glasgow

Black was Cullen's most distinguished student (pp.17 and 18). His discoveries in chemistry and physics have earned him a special place in the history of science. Black, like his mentor, achieved fame as a teacher. One of his students, who had attended his lectures in 1796, became Lord Chancellor and almost fifty years later wrote: 'I have heard the greatest understandings of the age giving forth their efforts in its most eloquent tongues – have heard the commanding periods of Pitt's majestic oratory – the vehemence of Fox's burning declamation – have followed the close compacted chain of Grant's pure reasoning . . . but I should without hesitation prefer, for mere intellectual gratification . . . to be once more allowed the privilege which I in those days enjoyed of being present while the first philosopher of his age was the historian of his own discoveries, and be an eye-witness of those experiments by which he formerly made them, once more performed with his own hands.' (Henry Brougham *Lives of men of letters and science who flourished in the time of George III*, London, 1845; 1: 348–9)

Black was also a prominent physician, whose patients included David Hume and other leading figures in the Scottish Enlightenment. In a description of his childhood, Sir Walter Scott wrote: 'I was an uncommonly healthy child but had nearly died in consequence of my first nurse being ill of a consumption, a circumstance which she chose to conceal, though to do so was murder to both herself and me. She went privately to Dr Black, the celebrated professor of chemistry, who put my father on his guard. The woman was dismissed and I was consigned to a healthy peasant . . .' (J.G. Lockhart *Memoirs of the life of Sir Walter Scott, Bart.* Edinburgh, 1837; 1:14).

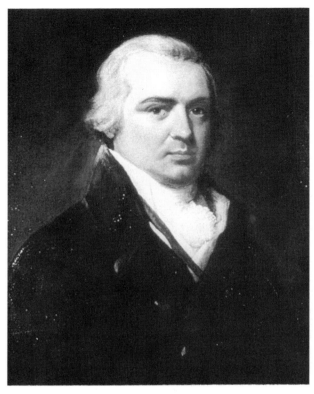

59. **Robert Willan** (1757–1812)   *Fig. 34*
General physician and dermatologist
Oil painting by an unknown artist
Colour photograph: Royal College of Physicians of London

Willan is often referred to as the founder of British dermatology.
During his student days in Edinburgh he came under Cullen's
influence and contributed to the proceedings of the Royal Medical
Society. Within ten years of graduation Willan produced an
outline of his plan for the arrangement and description of skin
diseases for which he was awarded the Fothergill medal of the
Medical Society of London. In his work *On cutaneous diseases*
(London, 1808) he presented an enlarged view of his nosology.

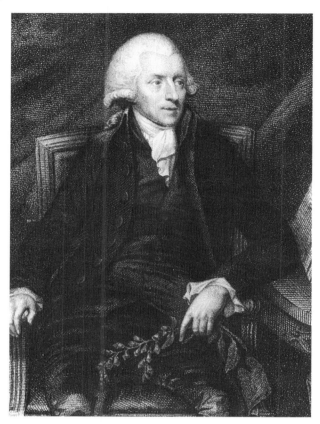

60. **William Withering** (1741–99)   *Fig. 35*
Botanist and physician
Engraving by W. Bond after C.F. von Breda

Withering's inspired investigation of the medicinal properties of
the foxglove was prompted by folk medicine. He spent ten years
recording its effects in cases of dropsy, noting particularly its value
when the pulse was irregular. His book *An account of the foxglove*
(Birmingham, 1785) is a medical classic which Cullen recommended
'should be in the hands of every practitioner of physic' (*Treatise of
the materia medica*, 1789; 2:555). During his student days in
Edinburgh, Withering said of Cullen: 'his affable disposition . . .
engages us in the pursuit of knowledge; his modesty is such that
whatever he advances as new he cautions us thoroughly to
examine, and only to embrace "with a slow-consenting academic
doubt" '.

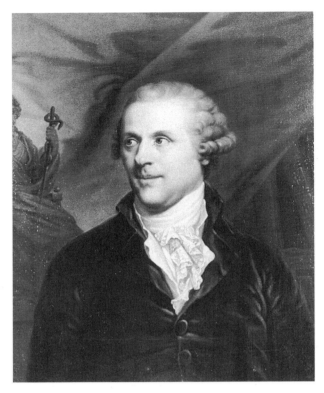

61. John Rogerson (1741–1823) *Fig. 36*
Physician to three Czars and Counsellor of State in Russia
Oil painting by J.G.B. Lampi
Photograph: Scottish National Portrait Gallery

Rogerson was physician to Catherine the Great and later to her son Paul and her grandson Alexander I. He became an adviser and close friend of the Empress and accompanied her on most of her travels, notably on her progress to the Crimea in 1787. Rogerson was an admirer of Cullen and corresponded with his former teacher, sending him descriptions of life in Russia.

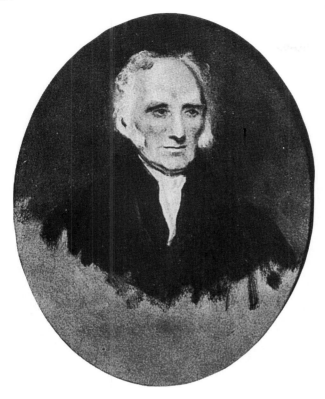

62. Sir Gilbert Blane (1749–1834)   *Fig. 37*
Naval physician
Oil painting by Sir Martin Shee
Photograph: Royal College of Physicians of London

As a student Blane attended courses of lectures given by William
Cullen, in Edinburgh, and William Hunter, in London. He was
personal physician to Admiral Sir George Rodney and Physician
to the Fleet. Through Blane's influence, the Royal Navy in 1795
adopted the recommendations, made by James Lind forty-two
years earlier, on the use of citrus fruit in the prevention of scurvy.
Blane did much to improve the living conditions of men in the
Navy.

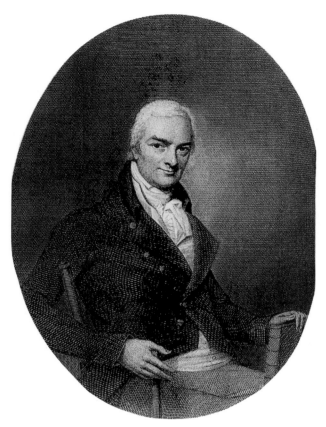

63. John Haygarth (1740–1827)   *Fig. 38*
Physician at Chester and Bath
Engraving by W. Cooke after J.H. Bell

Haygarth was a pioneer in the epidemiology, prevention and
control of infectious disease. At Chester Hospital he introduced
separate fever wards, the first example of the use of isolation in the
control of infectious disease in hospital. In 1793 he published his
*Sketch of a plan to exterminate the casual smallpox from Great
Britain and to introduce general inoculation*, an ambitious plan
which was far ahead of its time. He submitted some of his early
work to Cullen for criticism. Cullen later returned the compliment
by inviting the remarks of his former student on his *First lines of
the practice of physic*.

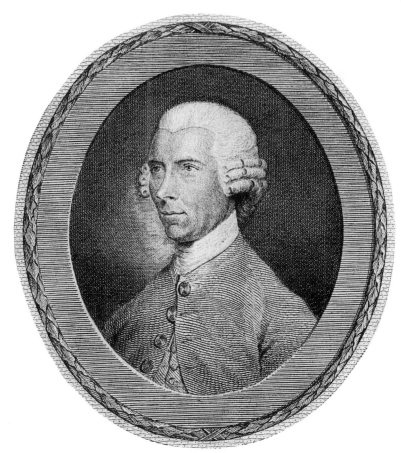

64. John Coakley Lettsom (1744–1813) *Fig. 39*
Physician and philanthropist
Drawing and engraving by T. Holloway
Thomson Walker Collection, TW1, L10
Photograph: Edinburgh University Library

Lettsom received part of his medical education in Edinburgh where Cullen's teaching stimulated his interest in fevers. He devoted much effort, as a Quaker, to the welfare of the poor among whom fevers were a major scourge. He championed the cause of vaccination against smallpox and played a prominent part in establishing the London system of dispensaries in an era when there were no hospital out-patient departments. He founded the London Medical Society in 1773. Lettsom's many benefactions were made possible by his wife's personal fortune and the rewards of a successful medical practice.

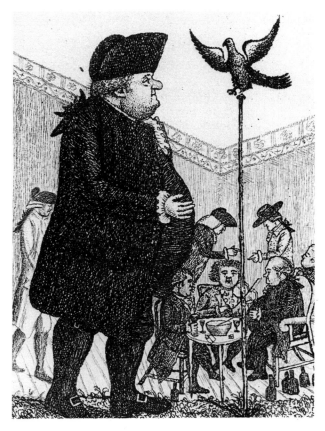

65. Dr John Brown (1735–88)   *Fig. 40*
John Kay *A series of original portraits*
2 vols, Edinburgh, 1837; 1
Photograph: Medical Illustration, University of Edinburgh

In this caricature of Brown he is represented with the ensign of the
Roman Eagle Masonic Lodge, which was carried before him as
Master of the Lodge in public processions. The scene in the
background depicts Dr Brown at a bowl of punch with some
friends. The two gentlemen in conversation, standing at the back
of this convivial group are Dr Cullen and his friend the professor
of midwifery, Dr Alexander Hamilton.

When Brown was a student Cullen recognised his merits as a
scholar and employed him as a tutor to his children. Brown later
became dissatisfied with the methods of medical treatment used by
Cullen and his professorial colleagues. He formulated a simple plan

of treatment based on his own theory of the causation of disease, which brought him into open conflict with Cullen and caused widespread and acrimonious debate especially in German medical schools. Several of Brown's views gained acceptance, but the most beneficial effect that he exercised on contemporary medicine was the discrediting of indiscriminate blood letting.

66. **John Brown** *Elementa Medicinae*
Edinburgh, 1780
Royal College of Physicians of Edinburgh

The Brunonian System, expounded in this work, attributed all disease to overstimulation or understimulation of the body; hence medical treatment had to be directed to stimulating the body or calming it. Brown's 'stimulants' included alcoholic beverages and opium.

67. **Dr James Graham** (1745–94)
The 'Prince of Quacks'
John Kay *A series of original portraits*
2 vols, Edinburgh, 1837; 1
Photograph: Medical Illustration, University of Edinburgh

Graham studied medicine at Edinburgh but did not graduate. He acknowledged publicly his indebtedness to Cullen, Monro, Black and others whose work he declared, had been of assistance to him in inventing and improving methods of treatment which possessed 'all the qualifications of the most perfect mode required by Celsus, of curing "*Cito, tuto & jucunde*," speedily, safely and agreeably.' Although some of Graham's ideas on hygiene were sensible most of his methods of treatment were those of a charlatan. After a tour of America, where he made a large amount of money he returned to London and set up his 'Temple of Health', in Adelphi. This was sumptuously furnished with a 'celestial bed' and fitted with immense mirrors, dragons breathing flames and electrical apparatus. Scantily dressed and nubile vestal virgins or goddesses looked after his patients.

68. **Lady Emma Hamilton** (1765–1815)
Lord Nelson's mistress
Oil painting by George Romney
Colour photograph: National Portrait Gallery, London

Emma Noble, before her marriage to Sir William Hamilton, is believed to have assisted Dr Graham in his Temple as a goddess of health.

Royal Medical Society

Cullen was an active supporter of this Edinburgh student society which encouraged critical debate in medicine, science and philosophy. As a student, he had attended the informal meetings which led to the foundation of the Society in 1737. He was elected an honorary member in 1764.

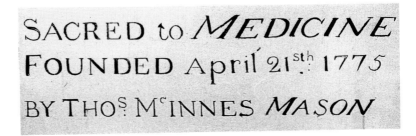

69. **Foundation Slab of the Royal Medical**   *Fig. 41*
Society's First Hall
Royal Medical Society
Photograph: Medical Illustration, University of Edinburgh

The slab covered the foundation stone. The following account is from the diary of a student officer-bearer of the Society: 'Was present at the laying of the foundation stone of a Hall for the Med. Soc. It was laid by our father of medicine, Dr Cullen, attended by . . . the whole Society; all the Professors . . . honored us with their company at supper. Old Cullen was very merry . . . we enjoyed ourselves more than we should have done at the great table. I stayed till about 2 in the morning.'
(*The Diary of Sylas Neville 1767–88*, ed. B. Cozens-Hardy, Oxford, 1950: 216).

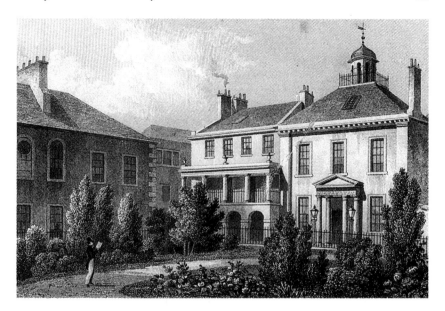

70. **Royal Medical Society Hall in Surgeons' Square**   *Fig. 42*
T.H. Shepherd *Modern Athens displayed in a series of views*
London, 1829
Photograph: Medical Illustration, University of Edinburgh

The Society's Hall is the building on the right with the weather vane. It was opened in 1776. In addition to the meeting room, the Hall contained a library and museum, and a chemical laboratory. This Hall continued in use until 1782 when it was sold to allow expansion of the old Royal Infirmary.

71. **Andrew Duncan** *Sen.* (1744–1828)
Physician
Oil painting by Sir Henry Raeburn
Colour photograph. Royal College of Physicians of Edinburgh

Duncan was a young extramural teacher when he advised that the Medical Society petition George III for a royal charter. This was granted in 1778.

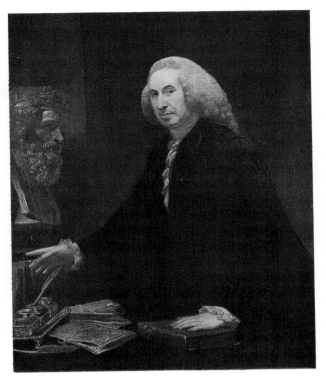

72. William Cullen (1710–90)   *Fig. 43*
Oil painting by David Martin
Royal Medical Society

This portrait was executed for the Royal Medical Society, in 1776, for its newly opened Hall. Dr Cullen's relatives regarded the likeness as exact as could be expected.

73. Joseph Black (1728–99)
Chemist and physician
Oil painting by David Martin
Colour photograph: Royal Medical Society

Cullen's former pupil and friend was painted for the Royal Medical Society as a companion to the portrait of Cullen by the same artist. It shows Black giving a lecture demonstration in chemistry.

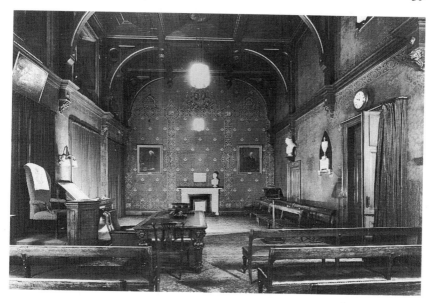

74. **Royal Medical Society Hall**   *Fig. 44*
in Melbourne Place
Photograph: Royal Medical Society

David Martin's companion portraits of Cullen and Black are seen
adorning the fireplace wall of the Society's second Hall. Both
portraits have been on loan to the Scottish National Portrait
Gallery since this Hall was demolished in 1965. The Society
celebrated its 250th anniversary in 1987 and continues to flourish
in its present home in the Student Centre near the Medical School.

Cullen's Edinburgh – the Old Town

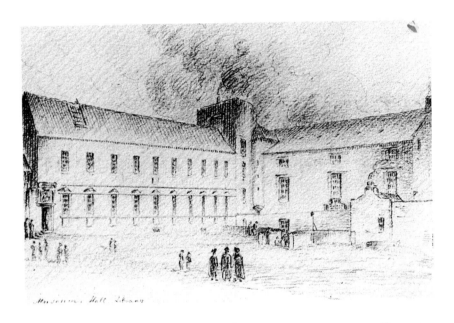

**75. Museum, Hall and Library of   *Fig. 45*
Edinburgh University**
Drawing by James Skene, 1817
Photograph: Edinburgh City Libraries

These were the principal buildings of Edinburgh University in the
eighteenth century. On the right is the Library where steps led
down to the Hall below. Many of the other buildings were in a
ruinous state.

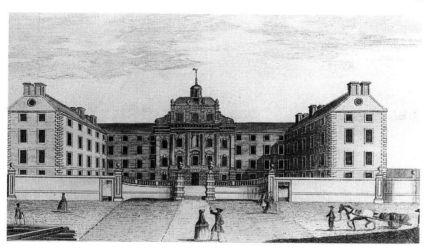

76. Edinburgh Royal Infirmary, *c.1746*   *Fig. 46*
Drawing and engraving by John Elphinstone
Photograph: Medical Illustration, University of Edinburgh

The first hospital, built on a U-shaped plan. It provided more light and better ventilation than the conventional European courtyard construction. When it was opened it was the finest public building in Scotland.

77. Detail of Map of Edinburgh   *Fig. 47*
in Mid-Eighteenth Century   overleaf
Compiled by Henry F. Kerr from Edgar's Plan
of 1742 and other sources (*Book of the Old
Edinburgh Club*, 1922; 11: 1–19)

The locations of Cullen's professional and social activities in the Old Town of Edinburgh are shown on this map.
1 College (University of Edinburgh)
2 Infirmary
3 Physicians' Hall
4 Mint (Cullen's home)
5 Nicolson's Tavern (in West Bow near junction with Cowgate)

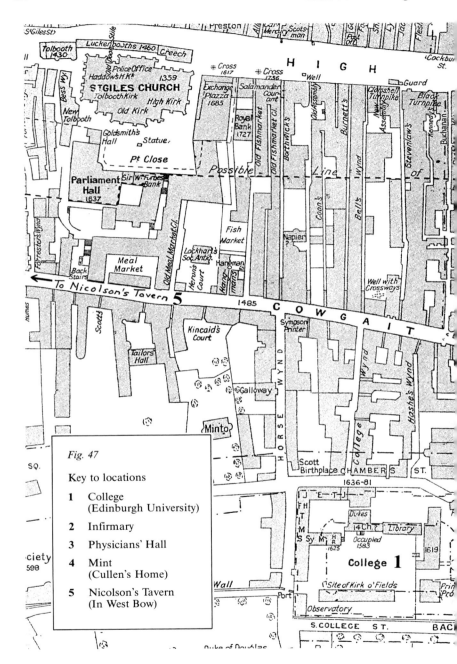

Fig. 47

Key to locations

1   College
    (Edinburgh University)

2   Infirmary

3   Physicians' Hall

4   Mint
    (Cullen's Home)

5   Nicolson's Tavern
    (In West Bow)

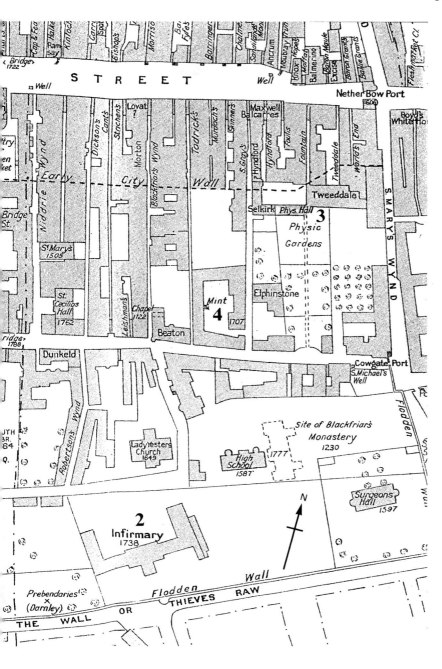

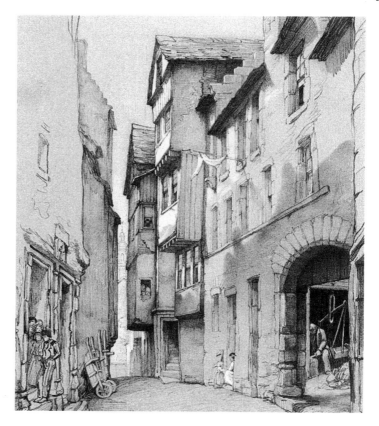

78. **Fountain Close**, site of the first Physicians' Hall   *Fig. 48*
Lithograph of drawing by James Drummond, 1833

This close lay between the High Street and the Cowgate. Its High
Street entrance remains, and is opposite John Knox's House. The
church, which may be faintly discerned at the foot of the close is
now St Patrick's Church and was built on the site previously
occupied by the College buildings. No picture of Physicians' Hall
in Fountain Close is known to exist.

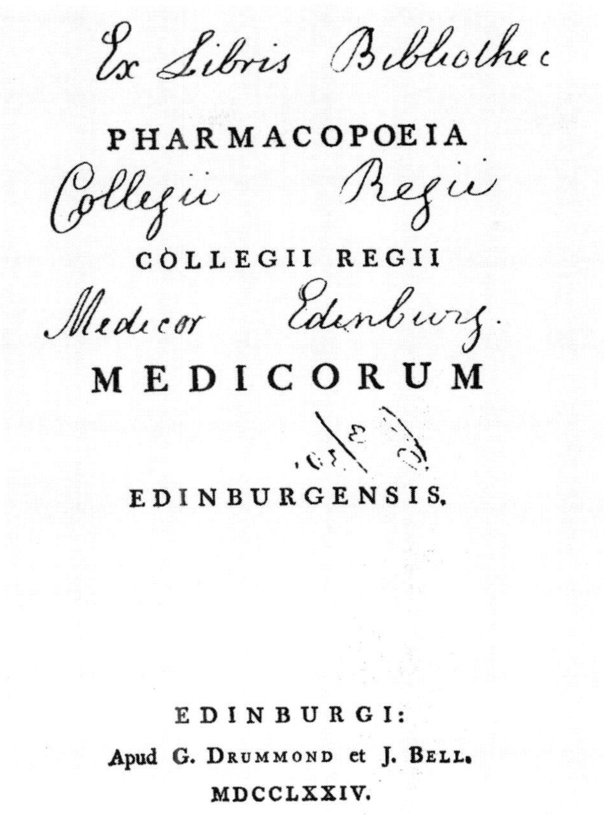

Ex Libris Bibliothec

PHARMACOPOEIA

Collegii Regii

COLLEGII REGII

Medicor Edinburg.

MEDICORUM

EDINBURGENSIS.

EDINBURGI:

Apud G. DRUMMOND et J. BELL,

MDCCLXXIV.

79. *Pharmacopoeia Collegii Regii*   *Fig. 49*
Medicorum Edinburgensis
6th edition, Edinburgh, 1774
Royal College of Physicians of Edinburgh

The 'Edinburgh Pharmacopoeia' had a major influence on drug prescribing. When the thoroughly revised and simplified 6th edition was issued, the President of the College, William Cullen, paid special tribute to the services given by Sir John Pringle in its preparation. After seven further editions the 'Edinburgh Pharmacopoeia' was replaced by the British Pharmacopoeia for national use in 1864.

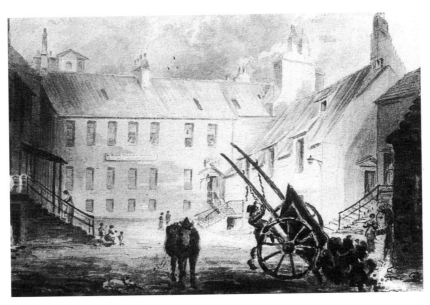

80. **William Cullen's House in Mint Court**   *Fig. 50*
Watercolour by James Skene, 1824
Colour photograph: Edinburgh City Libraries

Cullen lived in the Cowgate in the Mint Court at South Gray's
Close when the Cowgate was a fashionable part of Edinburgh. His
house is in the centre of the picture. It was built in the reign of
Charles II for the Master of the Mint and was known as the Earl
of Argyll's House because it was the lodging of the 9th Earl during
his attendance on the Scottish Parliament. This picture was
painted in the 19th Century when the house was occupied by a
lace-maker whose name board is affixed below the top row of
windows.

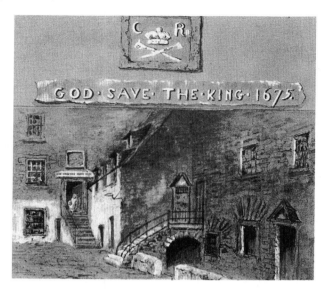

81. Entrance to Dr Cullen's House in Mint Court   *Fig. 51*
Watercolour by J. Stewart Smith
Colour photograph: City of Edinburgh Art Centre

The sculptured tablet above the doorway is decorated with the royal initials C.R.II, surmounting a crown with the inscription and date, GOD SAVE THE KING, 1675. This property was demolished in 1877.

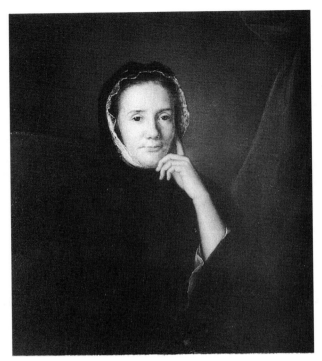

82. Mrs William Cullen   *Fig. 52*
Oil painting by William Cochrane
Colour photograph: Hunterian Art Gallery,
University of Glasgow

Mrs Cullen was the admiration and delight of all who met her. At
her home she entertained many of Cullen's students who appreciated her kindness and her fascinating and elegant conversation.
The Cullens had seven sons and four daughters. Mrs Cullen died in
1786, four years before her husband.

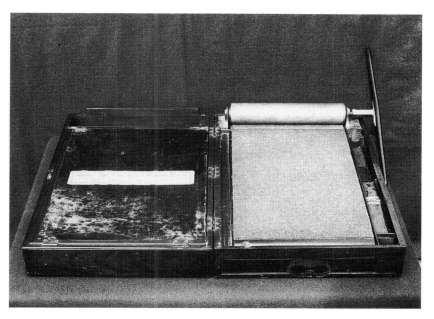

83. **Eighteenth Century Copying Machine**   *Fig. 53*
Invented by James Watt
Heriot-Watt University, Edinburgh

Cullen was among the first to use this machine. It was installed in his home where he dealt with his clinical correspondence. The machine was patented by Watt in 1780 and became standard office equipment for the next hundred years. The letter to be copied was written in a special ink, which Watt also invented. A blank page of thin, moistened paper was pressed upon it, and the resulting mirror image read through the paper. The portable machine on display was an original roller copying press and writing desk combined.

In the way of Medecine I advise him to take half
a muchkin of Lime Water every morning and an hour or
half an hour before dinner and again between seven and eight at night
Let him take the Tincture and Drops ordered below. The Tincture and
Drops are to be taken for a fortnight together and no longer.
They must be then laid aside for a fortnight at least and he
should only return to them when any accident has brought
back his complaints. The moderate Use of these Medecines
may be of Service but the long continued use of them would
do harm. Edr 26 Nov. 1768. William Cullen
℞ Cort. Peruv. cont. ℥ß Aurant. ℥j Canell. alb. ʒj Contusis affunde Aq.
bull. ℔j Macera per noctem & colaturæ adde Tinct. Cort. Peruv. ℥iv. Signa
Stomachic Tincture two table spoonfulls for a dose twice a day
℞ Tinct. Mart. ℥iß Aromat. ℥ß M Sig. Strengthening Drops thirty to be
taken in half a gill of water after every dose of the Tincture
W. C.

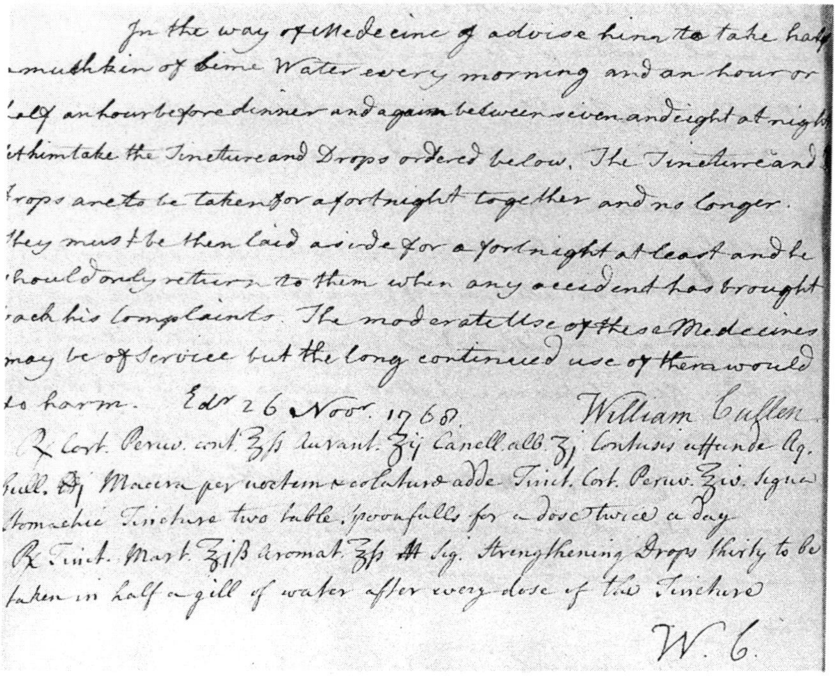

84. **Copies of Cullen's Letters** *Fig. 54a*
Royal College of Physicians of Edinburgh, (handwritten)
Cullen MSS 30, vols. 1 and 14

Cullen dictated letters to his amanuensis at home. Before despatch a handwritten copy of each letter was made for future reference. After 1 April 1781 James Watt's copying machine was used for this purpose. Examples are shown of copies made by hand (Fig. 54a, above) and by machine (Fig. 54b, opposite).

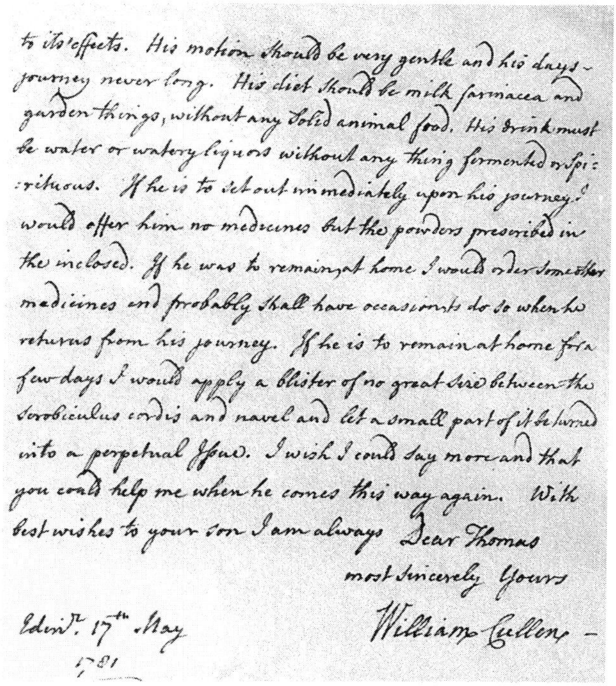

to its effects. His motion should be very gentle and his days journey never long. His diet should be milk farinacea and garden things, without any solid animal food. His drink must be water or watery liquors without any thing fermented or spirituous. If he is to set out immediately upon his journey I would offer him no medicines but the powders prescribed in the inclosed. If he was to remain at home I would order some other medicines and probably shall have occasion to do so when he returns from his journey. If he is to remain at home for a few days I would apply a blister of no great size between the scrobiculus cordis and navel and let a small part of it be turned into a perpetual Issue. I wish I could say more and that you could help me when he comes this way again. With best wishes to your son I am always *Dear Thomas*

most Sincerely Yours

William Cullen –

Edinr. 17th May
1781

Fig. 54b
(machine-made)

85. **James Watt** (1736–1819)

Engineer and scientist
Engraving by C.E. Wagstaff after W. Beechey
Photograph: Medical Illustration, University of Edinburgh

It was through James Watt's close friend, Joseph Black, that Cullen first learned of Watt's copying process. Watt was informed by Black that William Cullen and Adam Smith were particularly interested in his discovery.

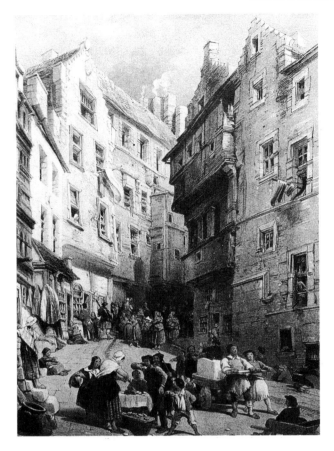

86. West Bow   *Fig. 55*
Lithograph by J.D. Harding after G. Cattermole

Cullen frequently retreated to Nicolson's Tavern in this part of the
town, where the notable company sometimes included Principal
Robertson, David Hume, Adam Ferguson and James Craig.

87. William Cullen
Drawing by an unknown artist
Thomson Walker Collection, TW1.C48
Photograph: Edinburgh University Library

The learned doctor 'todlen hame'.

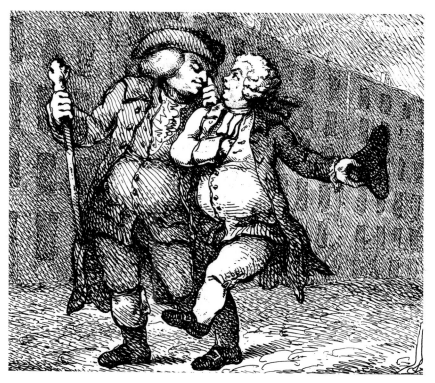

88. **Johnson and Boswell 'Walking up the High Street'**   *Fig. 56*
Etching by Samuel Rowlandson after designs
by Samuel Collings
Photograph: Medical Illustration, University of Edinburgh

In 1773 when Dr Johnson visited Edinburgh he was shown the
sights of the town and was introduced to James Boswell's circle of
friends. On Monday 16 August the great man visited the University
and the Royal Infirmary. Dr Cullen and his advocate son were
among the five guests invited to supper that evening to meet
Johnson. Cullen 'talked in a very entertaining manner of people
walking and conversing in their sleep.'

Cullen's Edinburgh – the New Town

Lord Provost Drummond's scheme to build a new town fired the enthusiasm of William Cullen, who strongly advocated that the new Hall of the College of Physicians should be built there.

The New Town was at first slow to develop because many did not believe that building on the lonely, windswept countryside to the north of Edinburgh would prove a successful venture. Confidence in the project had also been shaken by the partial collapse in 1769, of the newly built North Bridge, which was the only link between the Old and the New Towns.

Cullen lived to witness the successful launching of the first phase of the New Town development and the erection of some of its notable buildings.

89. North Bridge from the Base of Calton Hill
Lithograph by T.M. Baynes

This bridge was completed in 1772. It spanned the valley of the Nor' Loch which had been drained twelve years previously leaving a treacherous bog. Cullen was familiar with the site of construction because it lay close to the dam of the loch where the Physic Garden was situated during the early part of his career in Edinburgh. The bridge continued in use until it was rebuilt in 1896–7.

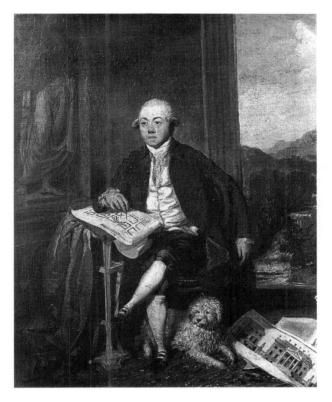

90. **James Craig** (1740–95) *Fig. 57*
Architect
Oil painting by David Allan
Colour photograph: Scottish National Portrait Gallery

James Craig's prizewinning plan was the basis for the development of the New Town. He designed and built the Physicians' Hall in George Street, which was his only important building in Edinburgh. In this portrait Craig is seen with a variant of his plan for the New Town. The drawing on the carpet shows his Physicians' Hall.

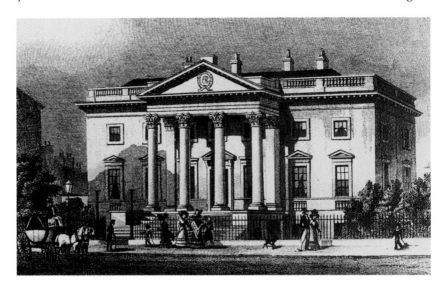

91. Physicians' Hall in George Street   *Fig. 58*
Designed by James Craig
T.H. Shepherd *Modern Athens displayed in a
series of views*, London, 1829
Photograph: Medical Illustration, University of Edinburgh

The foundation stone of this Hall was laid by William Cullen in
November 1775 during his Presidency of the College. In the
nineteenth century the Physicians decided to build a Hall more
suited to their needs and, in 1844, sold their expensive George
Street Hall to the Commercial Bank of Scotland.

92. Medals deposited in the Foundation
Stone of the Physicians' Hall in George Street
Royal College of Physicians of Edinburgh

After demolition of the Hall in 1844 two silver medals were found
in a glass bottle embedded in the foundation stone. One is gilded
and bears the motto 'Arti Salutiferae Sacrum' with engravings
depicting the George Street Hall and the Aesculapian serpent and
rod; the reverse is inscribed: 'Aedes Coll. Reg. Med. Edinb. – Hic
Positae XXVII Nov. A.D. MDCCLXXV – Curante Praeside
Gulielmo Cullen – Architecto Jac. Craig'.

The other medal bears the motto and the coat of arms of the City of Edinburgh; the reverse is inscribed: 'Jacobo Craig Architecto Propter Optimam Edinburgi Novi Ichnographiam – D.D – Senatus Edinburgensis – MDCCLXVII'.

93. Baron Ord's House in Queen Street

Designed by Robert Adam, 1770
Photograph: Royal College of Physicians of Edinburgh

This was one of the first notable houses in the New Town. It was bought by the Royal College of Physicians in 1864.

94. First Drawing Room in Baron Ord's House

Colour photograph: Royal College of Physicians of Edinburgh

In this room Baron Ord entertained David Hume, Adam Smith and other figures of the Scottish Enlightenment. It is now one of the Cullen Rooms in the College.

95. Sir Laurence Dundas' House

Designed by Sir William Chambers, 1772
T.H. Shepherd *Modern Athens displayed in a series of views*, London, 1829
Photograph: Medical Illustration, University of Edinburgh

This magnificent mansion, which stands on the east side of St Andrew Square, was bought by the Royal Bank of Scotland in 1825.

96. Register House in Princes Street

Designed by Robert Adam. Foundation stone laid, 1774
T.H. Shepherd *Modern Athens displayed in a series of views*, London, 1829
Photograph: Medical Illustration, University of Edinburgh

Houses the National Records in possibly the finest classical building in Edinburgh.

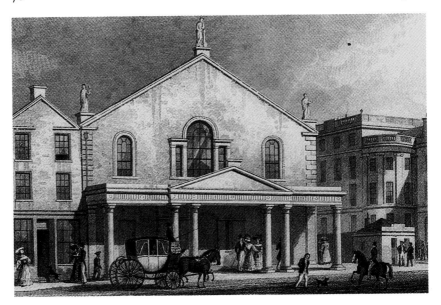

97. Theatre Royal   *Fig. 59*
Commissioned by David Ross, 1768
T.H. Shepherd *Modern Athens displayed in a
series of views*, London, 1829
Photograph: Medical Illustration, University of Edinburgh

The theatre stood on the site now occupied by the General Post
Office and was one of the first public buildings in the New Town.
The Kirk disapproved strongly of theatrical performances but in
1784 Mrs Sarah Siddons came to act in the Theatre Royal during
the sitting of the General Assembly of the Church of Scotland.
The Reverend Alexander Carlyle noted that the important business
of the Assembly had to be timed to allow the delegates to see the
famous actress perform.

Biography

98. John Thomson *An account of the life,*
lectures and writings of William Cullen MD
2 vols, Edinburgh, 1859

Some twenty years after Cullen's death his surviving family invited John Thomson to write this biography. Most of Thomson's information was obtained from written sources because he had not been personally acquainted with Cullen and death had removed those who had known him in his early career. Cullen's papers were made available to Thomson by his family and are now in the manuscript collections of the Royal College of Physicians of Edinburgh and the University of Glasgow. The first volume of the *Life*, published in 1832, was reissued with the second volume in 1859. The author was assisted by his eldest son, Dr William Thomson, both of whom died before the completion of the second volume. The work was concluded by Dr David Craigie.

99. Edward M. McGirr *William Cullen, MD (1710–1790):*
Cullen in context
Glasgow, 1990

In this review of Cullen's life and times his contributions to medicine and science are re-examined in the light of knowledge in the eighteenth century. The text of the booklet is based on a Stevenson Lecture in Citizenship, delivered by Professor McGirr during the bicentenary year of Cullen's death and the year in which Glasgow was designated European City of Culture.

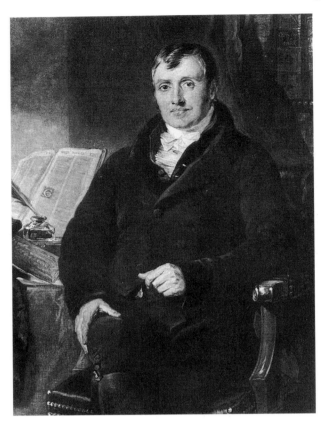

100. **John Thomson** (1765–1846)   *Fig. 60*
Surgeon and pathologist
Engraving by T. Hodgetts after Andrew Geddes

Cullen's principal biographer was the first professor of pathology
in the University of Edinburgh. He had previously held the posts
of professor of surgery in the Royal College of Surgeons of
Edinburgh and professor of military surgery in Edinburgh
University.

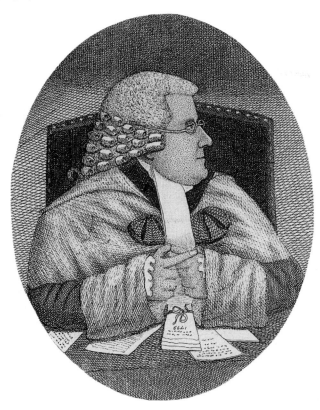

101. **Lord Cullen** (1742–1810)   *Fig. 61*
Senator of the College of Justice
John Kay *A series of original portraits*
2 vols, Edinburgh, 1838; 2

Dr Cullen's eldest son, Robert, possessed considerable literary
ability and made it known that he would write his father's
biography. Unfortunately posterity was deprived of this intimate
portrait. No such biography issued from the pen of the judge.

Remembrances

102. **Dr William Cullen** (1710–90)   *Frontispiece*
Oil painting: contemporary replica of portrait by William Cochrane
Royal College of Physicians of Edinburgh

Cullen was 58 when he sat for his portrait at the request of his students who wished to obtain engraved copies of the likeness of their great teacher. (The engraving was made by Valentine Green from which prints were published in 1772 by Thomas Sommers of Edinburgh.) The original painting is in the Scottish National Portrait Gallery and this replica was presented to the College in 1863 by Cullen's great-granddaughter, Mrs Marion Marjoribanks. It has been suggested that the copy was painted by Cochrane himself or at least under his supervision (L. Jolley, 'A note on the portraiture of William Cullen', *Bibliotheck* 1956–8; 1, no 3: 27–36).

103. **Dr Cullen's Gold-Headed Cane**
Royal College of Physicians of Edinburgh

In the eighteenth century the gold-headed cane was a symbol of the physician's social standing. This cane which was regularly used by Cullen is now one of the insignia of the Vice-President.

104. **Benjamin Rush** *An eulogium in honor of the late Dr William Cullen . . . delivered before the College of Physicians of Philadelphia, on the 9th July, agreeably to their vote on the 4th of May, 1790*
Philadelphia, 1790
Royal College of Physicians of Edinburgh

A tribute to William Cullen's achievements paid by one of his most distinguished former American pupils.

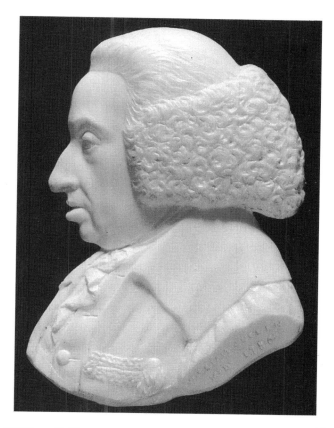

105. William Cullen   *Fig. 62*
Paste medallion by James Tassie
Royal College of Physicians of Edinburgh

This medallion, though dated 1786, is after a drawing of Cullen
by David Allan, 1774. Also on display was another version of this
medallion dated 1786. It is slightly larger and was cast in plaster.
Cullen is similarly attired in both medallions but his face shows
fewer signs of ageing in the larger version.

106. William Cullen's Grave and its enclosure at the burial
ground in the village of Kirknewton, Midlothian
Colour photograph: Royal College of Physicians of Edinburgh

The physician's memorial stone is above the entrance to the
enclosure and is surmounted by a medallion bearing his portrait.

THE SYMPOSIUM

I

William Cullen in eighteenth century medicine

CHRISTOPHER CLAYSON

President, I thank you for the honour you do me in inviting me to take part in this symposium. I appreciate the compliment highly and am most grateful to you. However, I have a second reason to be grateful. In the year 1752 William Cullen gave advice on the subject of retirement. He said 'A man retiring from the hurry of business, if he sit down entirely without employment, is apt to become uneasy and splenetic, and very ready to fall into amusements that are either trifling or hurtful to health'.[1] President, in beckoning me from the cool shades of retirement you have ensured that I have not been overtaken by the perils referred to by Dr Cullen.

In the latter half of the eighteenth century Edinburgh became the centre of that splendid flourish of learning, involving almost every human insight and activity, known as the Scottish Enlightenment. Among the members of this remarkable movement were three particular friends, Adam Smith, David Hume and William Cullen. Others involved were Joseph Black, Cullen's one time pupil and his successor in the chair of chemistry in Edinburgh; Adam Ferguson, now regarded as the founder of sociology; William Robertson, the Scottish historian; James Hutton, the founder of modern geology; Robert Adam and James Adam, the famous architects; Lord Monboddo and Lord Kames (Law Lords) and a dozen or so more. They met together for their lively discussions as members of various clubs. Almost all belonged to the Select Society founded by Allan Ramsay the painter. David Hume loved clubs where, he said, philosophers were ambassadors from the dominions of learning to those of conversation. The Reverend 'Jupiter' Carlyle, minister of Inveresk, had a slightly more pungent view. A virtue of the Select Society was that their discussions made the literati of Edinburgh less captious and pedantic than they were elsewhere. From this I infer that these clubbable people who made Edinburgh a 'hotbed of genius' were not averse to lively repartee which must have been a fruitful intellectual interchange among gifted men.[2]

The three members of the Scottish Enlightenment, Smith, Hume and

Cullen, whom I referred to as being particular friends encountered each other in connection with academic affairs in Glasgow, and it is to the West of Scotland therefore that I turn in order to introduce William Cullen.

He was born in Hamilton on 15 April 1710 and was educated at the local school. He went to Glasgow University where his attraction to medicine began, spurred on by an apprenticeship with Dr John Paisley, a surgeon. After a year or two spent in London and visiting the West Indies as a ship's surgeon, he returned to Scotland. From 1734–36 while in his early twenties he studied medicine more purposefully at Edinburgh University which was the only university in Scotland with an organised programme of medical teaching in a Faculty of Medicine. As a student he was a founder member of what became the Royal Medical Society. In 1736 Cullen returned to Hamilton where he set up practice and where a certain William Hunter became his resident pupil and partner. They worked together for three years till, on Cullen's advice, Hunter decided to seek his fortune in London. Cullen became a Doctor of Medicine of Glasgow University in 1740 and transferred his practice to the town in 1744. At the University he lectured in chemistry, botany (in Latin), materia medica and the practice of physic. He must have had an enormous capacity for work. Clearly his aim was to develop the rather rudimentary school of medicine in Glasgow into the more advanced type of school he had seen in Edinburgh as a student. He persuaded the authorities to provide him with a laboratory where he developed his experimental work in chemistry, and the connection of chemistry with agriculture.

Cullen has been referred to as founder of the Glasgow Medical School[3] to which he was appointed professor of medicine in 1751. A few days after his appointment to the chair of medicine Adam Smith was installed in the chair of logic and 'these two eminent men, each pursuing with indefatigable ardour his own branch of study, soon conceived a great esteem for one another and continued ever after to live in habits of most friendly and intimate intercourse.'[4] Very soon Smith was transferred to the chair of moral philosophy. David Hume, who had already published the third volume of his *Treatise on Human Nature*, was a candidate for the vacant chair of logic but the active support of both Cullen and Smith was not enough to overcome the Church's dislike of Hume's scepticism and he was unsuccessful. However all three remained close friends and their friendship was to be fortified in Edinburgh years later.

Late in 1755 Cullen was appointed professor of chemistry in Edinburgh. Since he had been professor of medicine in Glasgow it is perhaps not surprising that within two years of coming to Edinburgh he began his clinical lectures, developing the earlier Rutherford pattern, in the Royal

Infirmary. He succeeded to the chair of the institutes of medicine in 1766 and finally, after sharing the chair of medicine with John Gregory for some time, became sole professor in 1773 at the age of 63. During these academic changes he served for eight years as Secretary of the Royal College of Physicians of Edinburgh, and as President for two years from 1773. In 1775 he gave up his famous clinical lectures in the Royal Infirmary in order to meet the increasing demands of his chair and also of his private practice. He continued in the chair of medicine till shortly before his death which took place in his house in the old Scottish Mint in Gray's Close on February 5, 1790.

At work in Edinburgh

Less than a year after coming to Edinburgh in early 1756 Cullen was elected to the Fellowship of the College of Physicians. Shortly afterwards the College published a new revision of its 'Edinburgh Pharmacopoeia'. Cullen displayed particular interest in this work, and became actively involved in the production of subsequent editions. This remarkable pharmacopoeia was first published in 1699 after many years of active preparation. No doubt the early editions contained much that was useful, but there were many vegetable preparations so complicated as to suggest that ignorance of treatment could be masked by complexity in prescribing. There were also animal preparations so repugnant that they could only have got there in the first place through the ignorance and superstition of credulous ancestors. It seems to have been thought that the more revolting and unpalatable the remedy, the more probable the cure.

Some improvement was achieved in the 1756 edition largely due to the exertions of Dr John Clerk and Sir John Pringle[5] and the College decided that much more serious editing was required. It was felt that 'a clear intelligent head, a mind unfettered by prejudice and guided by firmness as well as knowledge' were needed for this task. Happily both Dr Cullen and Sir John Pringle possessed these qualities and, with the help of Joseph Black, they made major contributions to the next edition.[6,7]

Cullen's views on polypharmacy were appropriate for this purpose. He always enjoined students and practitioners to avoid complicated prescribing since they could not then decide which ingredient among several could have contributed to the patient's progress. Not surprisingly therefore the edition of 1774 showed enormous changes. By the time Cullen had completed his task in the 1783 edition the cobwebs, vipers, toads, snails, excrements, powdered skulls and the rest had gone. The break with the past which Cullen had helped to bring about confirmed the worth and fame of the Edinburgh Pharmacopoeia which was to endure till the British Pharmacopoeia was produced in 1864.

While it was one thing to reject bizarre treatments based on ancient superstitions, it was different dealing with a widely held opinion which had some slight smack of logic and even a whiff of theology. There was a belief, which Cullen seems to have shared, that in dying what was called the vital principle lingered in the body for some time after heart beat and respiration had stopped, and that this applied especially to the 'moving fibres' of the intestinal tissue. It was thought sometimes to be possible to stimulate the moving fibres, restore the vigour of the vital principle, and so encourage the patient's recovery.

This was the accepted thinking on which Cullen had to advise the President of the Board of Police in Scotland regarding the resuscitation of persons apparently drowned.[8] Cullen gave instructions about keeping the victim warm, and on the restoration of breathing. He then turned to the reactivation of the moving fibres in the intestine. For this a particular apparatus was required. It had essentially four parts, a combustion box, two tubes one from either side of the box, and bellows. Tobacco was ignited in the box. One tube was inserted into the subject's rectum, and the other was attached to the bellows. Tobacco smoke was then blown by the bellows into the intestinal canal – for two hours if necessary.

Today all this seems very strange. Yet I cannot help feeling that had I been there 200 years ago, armed only with the knowledge available to Cullen, I would have done exactly the same.

The advancement of knowledge

I am not the first to suggest that there are, especially as applicable to our profession, three phases in the advancement of knowledge. First, there is the observation of facts; second the hypothesis or reasoning to explain the facts; and third, there is the stage of subjecting hypothesis to absolute demonstration, or if you will, experimental proof.

In the drowning problem to which I have just referred experimental proof of the theory of resuscitation certainly did not emerge. Cullen was not an experimental physiologist in the Harveian sense. I think he, as a teacher of medicine, was very much more concerned with the ancient division which had separated the medical profession into those who were content with the observation of facts and those who also sought explanations. In medical history these two factions were called Empirics and Dogmatists.[9]

The empirics were satisfied with experience based on the accumulation of repeatedly observed facts. They treated symptoms rather than diseases. Similar symptoms received similar treatment even if due to different causes which the empirics did not inquire into too closely. What I have referred to as stage one of the advancement of knowledge was enough and they saw no need for anything more.

The dogmatists also respected facts but went further and sought explanations. This led to disentangling various disorders which could cause similar symptoms. In other words it meant attempting the classification of the 'natural shocks that flesh is heir to.' Several attempts in Europe had been made to do this before Cullen wrote his famous *Synopsis Nosologiae Methodicae*. The dogmatists utilised stage two of the advancement of learning, but had little idea of going further and subjecting their ideas to experimental proof although Cullen himself pointed to the value of hypothesis in leading to the discovery of more facts.[10]

It seems surprising to us today that the division between empirics and dogmatists lasted so long or indeed arose at all. Cullen however saw clearly that rational medicine must prevail and planned his teaching to that end.

He began the process in his clinical lectures which were clear, lively and entertaining.[11] He discussed with his students the history of the patient's symptoms and their significance for treatment. Clinical examination as we know it did not figure largely in their discussions. Percussion and auscultation were as yet unknown. He felt the pulse, assessed its quality and measured the rate by his sandglass.[12] He paid little attention to body temperature. The inaccurate thermometers were one foot long and the time required to take the body temperature was twenty minutes.[13] Cullen's pupil George Fordyce[14] trusted the patient's feelings more than thermometers in assessing body temperature. At suitable intervals Cullen reviewed the patient's progress and discussed with the class any therapeutic changes that were necessary. When the disease ended fatally and if he could obtain a post-mortem, he carefully went over the findings with them especially if the results showed that their professor had been clinically mistaken and 'the frivolity of his conjectures and practice discovered.'[15] All this was of course based on morbid anatomy. The concept of cellular pathology was still eighty years distant.

Later, as professor of medicine it was his custom annually in the first lecture of the systematic course to describe the way in which 'dogmatic' thought and practice must inevitably encompass the 'empiric'. He would discuss the disease classification in terms of his own nosological structure and look for the proximate cause (relevant to treatment) and the remote cause (relevant to prevention) but all, he said, based on facts and avoiding deductions of reasoning and hypotheses.

Cullen repeated these ideas in the preface to *First Lines of the Practice of Physic*[16] and stressed once more his intention to shun theories and hypotheses. It is this oft restated determination to avoid hypotheses which I find puzzling especially in view of his acknowledgement that hypotheses lead to the discovery of more facts. It is almost as if he regarded deductions of reasoning as established facts which required no proof. 'The facts of physic are more frequently the inference of reason than the simple objects of sense.'[17] Reading his work today it seems as if he were advancing hypotheses all the time, and indeed nowhere more clearly than in the *First Lines*. He stated that the remote causes of small pox, measles, plague, mumps, leprosy and 'diseases of venery' (but strangely enough, seldom tuberculosis) were specific contagions. Continuing fever and intermittent fever were similarly caused, the contagious matter in the former coming directly from human beings and in the latter indirectly from marsh miasmata.[18] To Cullen this was not hypothesis. David Hume might have said that he was inferring the unobserved cause from the observed result. To us the reasoning was entirely plausible but still only hypothesis. Yet we should remember that only one man had gone further than Cullen in advancing an hypothesis on the actual nature of contagious matter. That was Benjamin Marten[19] who suggested that all these disorders, together with some diseases of animals were caused by 'certain *species* of Animalcula or wonderfully minute living Creatures, that by their peculiar Shape or disagreeable Parts, are inimical to our Nature; but however capable of subsisting in our Juices and Vessels.' But all this theory was only stage two in the advancement of the knowledge of contagion. Stage three, the proof, had to wait for another hundred years. I do not think that the experimental proof of hypotheses was so much in Cullen's mind. He was rather more concerned that after centuries of divergence he would see the empirics amalgamated with the dogmatists, or as he preferred it with the rationalists. He disliked the implication of the word 'dogmatist'. He said 'Every wise physician is a dogmatist but, a dogmatical physician is the most absurd animal that lives', and 'I profess to be a dogmatist but I should be very sorry if any person thought me dogmatical'.[20] His friend David Hume would have liked that. So successful was Cullen in merging empiric with dogmatic practice that by the time his successor James Gregory was in the chair of medicine the word 'empirics' was virtually reserved for quacks.[21]

The pirated lectures

When Dr Charles Alston, professor of medicine and botany, died in late 1760 shortly after commencing the course of lectures which he regularly gave in materia medica, Cullen was called on to finish the task. Eleven years later he was distressed to learn that a volume had been published in London entitled *Lectures on the Materia Medica as delivered by William Cullen, M.D., Professor of Medicine in the University of Edinburgh*.[22] What had happened was that two of his students in 1761 had taken full notes and decided to publish not for monetary benefit but to ensure a wider circulation of Cullen's ideas. As they said in their preface 'The Editors have no other motive for making this Work public, than a concern to find a Performance, which so far excells in method, copiousness of thought, liberality of sentiment and judgement, all that have been before written on the subject, in danger of being lost to the world'.

Not surprisingly Cullen was angry so far as such a charitably disposed man could be. He had not revised his notes of 1761 which were merely the basis of lectures delivered as a stand-in for Dr Alston. He felt that the lectures delivered without notes would inevitably fall short of the written standards required for publication. Again, when published they were eleven years out of date implying that he, Cullen, had made no progress in materia medica during that period.

We can understand Cullen's annoyance. He applied to the London High Court of Chancery for an injunction to stop the sale, and this was immediately granted. When however it was represented to him that a great many copies were already in circulation, Cullen agreed to the sale of the remainder on condition that he would receive a share of the profits, and that the grosser errors in the work should be corrected. Furthermore it is clear that he insisted on a new title page and an additional preface for the remaining unsold copies in order to make his stated anxieties about the volume clear.[23] This was done and the second preface concluded as follows. 'They [the editors] hope that they have done enough to show what might be expected from the accuracy of the Author's own hand . . . but they are assured by himself that his other occupations, and time of life, make it very probable that he never will engage in it.'

They were all wrong, and Cullen set to work. His expanded and more authoritative *Treatise of the Materia Medica* was finally published in 1789. As compared with the lectures pirated by his students a more scientific approach became obvious. In the Treatise he repeatedly seems to ask three questions. What is the immediate aim of treatment; what is the action of medicine; and what is the result? We can hardly better that plan today.

The sale of medical degrees

In the eighteenth century medical impostors were a considerable problem. It seems that a would-be practitioner who posted his fee could obtain a doctorate in physic without attending classes or presenting himself for examination.[24] This was not permitted in Edinburgh but was commonplace in the Universities of St Andrews and Aberdeen, and even the University of Glasgow was not above suspicion. Therefore the possession of a doctorate was no guarantee that its owner was knowledge-able. In 1754 William Hunter wrote to his old chief from London informing him that the practice of selling degrees was doing Scotland's medical reputation much harm.[25] Although Cullen was professor of medicine in Glasgow at the time I cannot find that he took any action. During his tenure of the chemistry chair in Edinburgh a dreadful lapse occurred in the University, hitherto the model of academic rectitude. An illiterate brushmaker in London, one Samuel Leeds, sent his fee and received a doctorate.[26]

However, in 1773 Cullen became not only sole professor of medicine but was also elected President of the Royal College of Physicians of Edinburgh. He offered the Honorary Fellowship of the College to the Duke of Buccleuch who was widely involved in public work and was a member of the House of Lords. The Duke wished most heartily that it would be in his power to show his gratitude and inquired about the selling of degrees and how such a pernicious practice could be stopped.[27]

This I imagine was Cullen's chance. He wrote a detailed Memorial on the subject and offered a solution which showed great foresight.[28] He recommended a system of visiting Royal Commissioners to inspect medical schools, and correct abuses, and further proposed a minimum period of two years' student training before examination which would be the only way to a degree.

Before taking the problem to the government, as Cullen had hoped, the Duke first sent the Memorial to Adam Smith for his opinion. We do not know what advice Adam Smith gave him but we do know what he wrote to his old friend Cullen.[29] It was a splendid piece of English prose with much friendly raillery. Clearly he thought that Cullen was making much ado about very little. 'Quacks' he said 'are too contemptible to be considered rivals. Do not all the old women in the country practice physic without exciting murmur or complaint? And if here and there a graduate doctor should be as ignorant as an old woman, where can be the great harm?' In summary the famous economist's views were that all should be allowed to practise medicine who chose to do so; Universities should not have a monopoly of teaching but there should be free and unfettered competition; and the selection of teachers may be most safely entrusted to students.

It seems that the Duke of Buccleuch took no further action and Cullen was disappointed. The situation demanded a powerful reply to Smith which came in his next graduation address.[30] It did not seem like friendly raillery. 'Those ignorant of the art . . . cannot judge the employment of the art.' 'In the practice of medicine, what ever may go on elsewhere none of the reasons for unfettered competition have any force.' 'It is essential that the title of Doctor of Medicine ensures that its owner is both learned and skilful.' 'In Edinburgh University the best regulations are faithfully observed to that end.'

All this eloquence, and more, had little effect and change came slowly. Ultimately however Cullen's sense of direction proved correct and the principles of the main recommendations in his memorial were incorporated, long after his death, in the Medical Act of 1858.

Moderation in the Enlightenment

William Cullen must have had a very pleasing personality. I am sure that he enjoyed lecturing. A professor does not lecture two to four hours a day five days a week[31] unless he is happy in his work, and we may conclude that he was a very good teacher. So much is manifest from the number of pupils he attracted from Europe and from America, many of whom in turn achieved fame in their own countries.

Yet Cullen was much more than a good lecturer. He was also a dedicated mentor. He made friends with his students, especially those who applied themselves. He invited groups of them to his home for supper and discussed with them not just medicine but also their interests and personal problems. If he found one to be in reduced circumstances he might contrive privately to waive his fee even though he was largely dependent on fees for his livelihood. From time to time he was called on to treat students who were ill and made no charge even though he was entitled to do so.

This generosity also extended to his patients. He treated the indigent and the prosperous without discrimination. If payment of fees were to cause embarrassment he did not press the claim. Indeed, 'to his patients his conduct . . . was so pleasing and his address so affable and engaging, his manner so open, so kind and so little regulated by pecuniary considerations . . . that he became the friend and companion of every family he visited.'[32]

Cullen's general approach to medicine fits well with this benevolent personality. The burden of his famous consultation letters indicates that balance and moderation in all human activities were essential. Moderate meals secure health and promote long life. In therapy he favoured only one drug at a time. He did not believe in polypharmacy. He usually advised only a little blood letting; occasionally it was preferable to give up meat.[33] Laxatives should be mild without purging; and emetics should generally stop short of 'full vomiting'.

Among the physicians of his time he identified two types of practitioners.[34] There were those who could and did cause mischief by being too bold and rash. On the other hand there were also others who, rather like the old empirics, far from being bold and rash left too much to nature. This produced caution and timidity which, he said, ever opposed the introduction of new and efficacious remedies.

He was not the first to describe this therapeutic dilemma between caution and boldness. A century before Cullen's time Sir Francis Bacon[35] drew attention to the same phenomenon. 'Physicians are some of them so pleasing and conformable to the Humour of the Patient, as they press not the Cure of the Disease. And some others are so Regular, in proceeding according to Art, for the Disease, as they respect not sufficiently, the condition of the Patient.' He wisely concluded 'summon a doctor of a middle Temper.'

I think William Cullen was indeed a doctor of the middle temper. And when you come to think of it, no greater compliment could be paid to this man of judgement who shaped eighteenth-century medicine in the way it was to go till the emerging study of cellular pathology opened up new knowledge in the nineteenth century.

Acknowledgements

It is a pleasure to acknowledge my great indebtedness to Miss Joan P.S. Ferguson MA, ALA, and Mr Iain Milne ALA for making the resources of the Library of the Royal College of Physicians available to me.

References

1. J. Thomson, *Life of William Cullen M.D.* (2 vols, Edinburgh 1859), vol. 1, p. 69.
2. D. Daiches, P. and J. Jones (eds), *A Hotbed of Genius* (Edinburgh 1986), pp. 35, 65.
3. D. Guthrie, *A History of Medicine* (Edinburgh 1945), p. 222.
4. Thomson, *Life*, vol. 1, p. 71.
5. C. Gordon, 'Sir John Pringle and the apothecaries', *Pharmaceutical Historian* 19 (1984), pp. 5–12.
6. Thomson, *Life*, vol. 2, pp. 81–4, 571–4.
7. D.L. Cowen, 'The Edinburgh Pharmacopoeia', in R.G.W. Anderson and A.D.C. Simpson (eds), *The Early Years of the Edinburgh Medical School* (Royal Scottish Museum, Edinburgh 1976), pp. 25–45.
8. W. Cullen, *A Letter to Lord Cathcart . . . concerning the recovery of persons drowned and seemingly dead* (Edinburgh 1774), pp. 12–14.
9. L.S. King, *The Medical World of the Eighteenth Century* (Chicago University Press 1958), pp. 31–58.
10. See R. Passmore, 'Method of Study. William Cullen. An introductory lecture to the course of the Practice of Physic given at Edinburgh University in the years 1768–89', *Proc. R. Coll. Phys. Edin.* 17 (1987), pp. 268–85.
11. Thomson, *Life*, vol. 1, pp. 107–10, 121.
12. H.G. Graham, *The Social Life of Scotland in the Eighteenth Century* (London 1899), vol 1. p. 116.
13. D. Guthrie, *History of Medicine*, p. 298.
14. W.F. Bynum, 'Cullen and the study of fevers in Britain, 1760–1820', in W.F. Bynum and V. Nutton (eds), *Theories of Fever from Antiquity to the Enlightenment* (Medical History, Supplement No. 1, 1981; London, Wellcome Institute for the History of Medicine), pp. 135–47.
15. Thomson, *Life*, vol. 1, p. 108.
16. W. Cullen, *First Lines of the Practice of Physic* (Edinburgh, new ed. in 2 vols, 1802), p. xxv.
17. M.B. Strauss (ed.), *Familiar Medical Quotations* (Boston 1968), p. 485.
18. Cullen, *First Lines*, vol. 1, pp. 75–82, 345–96, 502.
19. B. Marten, *A New Theory of the Consumptions* (London, 1720), p. 51.
20. Thomson, *Life*, vol. 1, p. 111.

21. King, *Medical World of the Eighteenth Century*, pp. 55–6.
22. [W. Cullen], *Lectures on the Materia Medica as delivered by William Cullen M.D.* (London 1772), p. iii.
23. *Ibid.* (1773 imprint), pp. vii-viii.
24. D. Hamilton, *The Healers* (Edinburgh 1981), p. 143.
25. Thomson, *Life*, vol. 1, p. 660.
26. *Ibid.*, pp. 462–5.
27. *Ibid.*, p. 467.
28. *Ibid.*, pp. 468–72.
29. *Ibid.*, pp. 473–81.
30. *Ibid.*, pp. 482–6.
31. R. Chambers and T. Thomson (eds), *A Biographical Dictionary of Eminent Scotsmen* (3 vols, Glasgow 1868–70), vol. 1, p. 410.
32. Thomson, *Life*, vol. 1, p. 121.
33. R. Stott, 'Health and Virtue: or, how to keep out of harm's way. Lectures on Pathology and Therapeutics by William Cullen c.1770', *Medical History* 31 (1987), pp. 123–42.
34. Cullen, *First Lines*, vol. 1, p. ix.
35. Quoted by G. Keynes in *The Life of William Harvey* (Oxford 1966), p. 159.

2

William Cullen and the practice of chemistry

J.R.R. CHRISTIE

Twenty years ago, very little was known or written concerning Cullen's chemical career. Since that time, Arthur Donovan's thorough treatment of Cullen's chemical doctrines, my own more narrowly focused work on his experimental and theoretical chemistry, Jan Golinski's studies of Cullen's chemical didactics and the public dimensions of his chemistry and Charles Withers' work on Cullen's scientific agriculture have produced a complex picture.[1] If twenty years ago Cullen was thought of as a gifted chemical teacher whose main contribution to chemistry was his illustrious pupil Joseph Black, and who maintained an interest in applied chemistry, we now have an immeasurably more interesting and significant characterisation. It is that of someone who effected major structural change in chemical teaching and in the image of chemistry which could be offered to a widening scientific and lay public; who aligned chemistry simultaneously with the epistemological programmes of his philosophical friends and colleagues and the civic and utilitarian goals of Enlightened Improvers; who navigated the tricky shoals of client-patron relations and academic politics with consistent success to make crucial moves in consolidating and advancing his career; who paid consistent and innovative attention to the applied chemistry of agriculture and bleaching; whose practical pedagogy was a highly self-conscious and critical development of contemporary and historical discursive traditions of chemical teaching; and who originated and pursued an ambitiously innovative and potentially far-reaching programme of experimental and theoretical research which, though unconsummated in the terms it set itself, was nevertheless of major significance in establishing the topics, problems and approaches which would typify much physico-chemical and medico-chemical research in Scotland into the 1780's.

By re-surveying and synthesising these findings, this essay attempts to give an overview of what the practice of chemistry and being a chemist involved at that time. It is apparent to anyone who works with Cullen's chemical papers, the best collection of which resides in the

Library of the Royal College of Physicians of Edinburgh, that Cullen's practice as a chemist cannot easily be sorted into neat and distinctly separate categories, of researcher, teacher, improver and so on. In my own attempts to reconstruct Cullen's academic chemical researches, I found myself most often using material found in the manuscript notes by students of his chemistry lectures, in the course of which, and only in the course of which, are to be found elaborated his more advanced notions in chemical theory.[2] Existing copies of such teaching notes across a period of years are what allow the historian to produce something of a developmental picture of Cullen's chemical theory. Again, to find Cullen's theoretical interpretation of some of his experimental research, one is obliged to read not the remnants we have of research papers, but the lecture notes which contain a generalised theoretical expression of Cullen's experimental conclusions.[3] Clearly, therefore, any distinction which we ourselves might make between, on the one hand, chemical teaching by lecture, and on the other, theoretical research, is inappropriate with respect to Cullen, and probably for other lecturing and teaching chemists at that time. Comparably, too, I note that Charles Withers' treatment of Cullen's agricultural science is able firstly to trace much of it back to his chemical teaching at both Glasgow and Edinburgh; and secondly, is able to make sense of Cullen's approach to agriculture primarily through the category of 'Philosophy'.[4] Again, if one is interested in establishing the development and range of Cullen's theoretical views on evaporation and solution, both central theoretical topics for him, one needs finally to follow them through to their use in Cullen's study of bleaching processes for the Board of Trustees.[5] Reciprocally, his work on common salt production has relevance for the understanding of his research on the classification of salts and the section of his lectures on salts.[6] Consequently any effort to synthesise the full range of Cullen's chemical practice will turn out to be something more interesting and challenging than a simple aggregate of distinct and separate activities. It has instead to be a form of integration, capable of spelling out the several significances of any given moment of chemical practice with respect to a variety of educational, social, technological and scientific contexts. Rarely with Cullen would it ever be a simple case of one thing at a time.

It is also apparent from the foregoing that the most central and consistent resource for historical research on Cullen's chemistry is the sequence of manuscript lecture notes we have remaining, which provide a reasonable, if partial, spread of them across his years as a chemist at both Glasgow and Edinburgh.[7] As already emphasised, they contain very substantial traces of his academic research and his applied chemical activities, to the extent that we can say that it was actually in the course of his chemical lecturing that he was able to develop his distinctive approach to agricultural science, to applied chemistry in general, and to highly generalised theories of the states of matter and chemical reactivity.

These lectures can also be understood as being informed by other substantial preoccupations and contexts. In Glasgow particularly, his auditors were not solely medical students, but students from other, non-medical classes, as well as non-registered, non-matriculating men 'engaged in any business connected with chemistry' (Dr Wallace).[8] Cullen's widely focused approach to chemical teaching was one he adopted from the outset of his lecturing career, and it was designed to have both intellectual and practical appeal to a diverse audience; students with general natural philosophical interests, as well as medical students; members of local mercantile and manufacturing communities; and men occupied with farms and landed estates, or who could expect in future to be so. One could go even further, to say that Cullen's two most important auditors were present in a virtual sense only. His chemical career from the outset was substantially indebted to the favour of Archibald Campbell (Lord Ilay, later the 3rd Duke of Argyll) and Henry Home (Lord Kames), both men of strong improving bent.[9]

It is too much to say that their patronage simply imposed certain applied chemical interests upon William Cullen. Equally there can be no doubt that Cullen's persistent attention to agricultural chemistry in his lectures at Glasgow, and later at Edinburgh, was due partly to Henry Home's continued requests for a treatise on agriculture from Cullen's pen.[10] Similarly, one ought to relate Cullen's devotion to problems of salt analysis and production less to any local Glasgow-based manufacturing interests, but more to the sea-going sector of the economy of Lord Ilay's West Coast estates.[11] To understand Cullen's assiduity on these matters in his lectures we need to realise first of all the pervasiveness of the client-patron relation with respect to the life of an individual such as Cullen. Favour from the great was not an event occurring now and then. It was conditional for most academic appointments and was a basis for career advancement. So long as political power took the personalised form it did in the eighteenth century, patrons such as Lord Ilay and Lord Kames were decisive in the disposal of legal appointments, clerical livings, university chairs and similar posts of influence. Their power was therefore ensured, maintained and extended. Under these conditions Cullen's relations with his patrons were of first importance when he harboured growing career ambitions to move to Edinburgh. Though these men were geographically removed, Cullen was always aware of their presence because of their power to affect the direction and prosperity of his life, and it is hardly surprising that their specific intellectual and economic interests were represented and developed in his lectures. He was able, however, to generalise the role of applied chemist to that of general chemical improver, demonstrating concern not only with salt production and agriculture but with a whole range of production which was dependent upon knowledge of chemical processes. This came in the latter half of his chemistry course, where he dealt with the five major heads of the classification of chemical substances, pointing out the manufacturing processes to which each class of chemical substances related.[12] Together with his specific attention to agricultural matters such as animal and vegetable chemistry, this aspect of Cullen's teaching allowed him to develop the public image of the chemist as improving citizen and the wielder of useful knowledge that would promote the material betterment of his community. This was done in a highly self-conscious fashion. Cullen, that is, did not just promote this image of the chemist simply as its exemplar, rather he conceptualised it for his students, by situating the labour of the chemical philosopher in relation to that of the merchant and the work of artisans. The merchant's work is entrepreneurial and managerial, to assess demand and marketing opportunity and to direct the work of the artisan. The chemical philosopher acts in the capacity of consultant, able to refine and improve manufacturing processes with the aid of his special analytical knowledge, not in any haphazard manner, but with specific regard to the discernment of the market made by the merchant.[13]

This orientated teaching of the improver-chemist's role of course contrasts notably with Cullen's own situation as a practical improver. He did not work on applied chemical topics discerned by Glaswegian entrepreneurs. His work on agriculture, particularly at Kames's prompting, on salt in the interest of Lord Ilay, and on bleaching in relation to the Board of Trustees, particularly Lord Deskford were at the request of legal, landed, titled men. In effect, therefore, we can say that the mercantile entrepreneurship envisaged by Cullen for his students as appropriate for the practice of improving chemistry, was displaced by the interests of a far more powerful group, the aristocrats and gentry and their cadets who owned the land of Scotland. Cullen could not but be aware of this. The specific targeting of merchants as key figures in his Glasgow lectures must therefore relate to the potential or actual presence of such men in his audience – a piece of local public relations work indicative of how important the precise context of Cullen's utterances were, if we are to understand all their nuances.

These improving interests form only a relatively minor, though not negligible portion of Cullen's chemical teaching. The substance overall of his course had most often a critical point of departure. Whether talking of previous definitions of chemistry, of particular chemical doctrines or analyses, Cullen would give his own appraisal which was frequently critical of others' inadequacies; Boerhaave, Stahl, Pott, Muschenbroek, Desaguliers – very few escaped unscathed.[14] Cullen retained formal discursive aspects of the European chemical lecturing tradition, encompassing history of chemistry, 'chemical instruments', definition of chemistry, chemical principles, and so forth; but his ordering of these categories (such as he thought proper to include within them, based on his views of the curricular function of chemistry at that time), all marked him out as a chemical pedagogue who was innovative and in certain respects radical.

In contrast with two major proponents of alternative European chemical traditions of thinking, Boerhaave and Macquer, Cullen did not initiate the main substance of his course by giving instruction on the theoretical principles of chemistry. He followed Boerhaave in having an historical introduction and in devoting space to what were called Instruments; meaning by that not what we mean, a test-tube or a furnace, but more generally those things and agents which the chemist most commonly and crucially deployed in his investigations.[15] In this sense for Boerhaave, fire or heat was an 'Instrument', as was water, in its role of a general solvent.[16] But he regarded the overall movement of Boerhaave's course, from theory to practice, as inadequate, and did not categorically feature a theoretical section as such in his lectures.[17]

This may make it sound as if Cullen had adapted existing continental didactic practice to the more severe Baconian and Newtonian methodological climate which prevailed in Britain. Other aspects of his presentation would indeed support this viewpoint, such as his overall emphasis on the definition of chemistry as a collection of factual knowledge, and his experimental-taxonomic approach to the study of salts and their properties. Paradoxical as it may appear, Cullen's chemistry course was much more speculative and theoretically inclined than those of contemporary British chemists such as Shaw, Dossie and Lewis.[18] What Cullen did was to abandon theory as a didactic category but include theory within the other didactic categories he retained. This is how we find theory recurring throughout the several sections of his lectures. His history of chemistry emphasised its appeal to the liberal and speculative mind; approaching the topic of heat he remarked, 'You must in this and other subjects indulge me in giving much Theory'.[19] And his treatment of chemical species, the salts, earths, inflammables etc., also introduced theoretical considerations.[20] Cullen's abandonment of the didactic category of theory therefore has to be considered as a formal departure from continental practice; but it did not entail any abandonment of theoretical content; his lectures appear decidedly speculative in tone when placed alongside those of the avowedly Baconian Peter Shaw.[21]

Cullen's justification for theory was threefold. Following Hume, and perhaps more specifically Adam Smith, he held that theoretical speculation was, from a psychological point of view, more or less unavoidable. More particularly, for the chemical enquirer theory had a powerful heuristic role to play; it was 'a most powerful means of exciting us to experiments'.[22] Finally, theory lent the practice of chemistry what he and contemporaries termed a 'liberal' cast. That is, it was the possession of theory which in large part transformed the very form of knowledge which chemistry constituted: transformed it from being a collection of factual knowledge largely related to arts such as pharmacy, agriculture, bleaching, sugar refining and salt making, into a philosophy or science, fit for inclusion in its own right in a university curriculum, and fit to form part of the instruction of gentlemen, rather than artisans.[23]

Cullen's devotion to chemical theory was in other words part of his effort to redesignate the social and educational status of chemistry and the public image of the chemist. His particular achievement here was to do it by bringing in the notion of philosophy, equating chemistry thereby with moral and natural philosophy in the liberal arts curriculum, but without selling out on the, for him equally necessary, component of improving, utilitarian, applied chemistry. Cullen had therefore undertaken a complex re-drawing of chemistry's relations in the academy and in the world. In summary form it was as follows. The philosophical chemist was philosophical in respect of possessing a comprehensively methodised approach to his field of knowledge, and in respect of his devotion to and command of theoretical knowledge. It was this theoretical knowledge that rendered him conversant with fundamental causal principles in nature, as the natural philosopher was conversant with physical phenomena and the moral philosopher, in his domain, had knowledge of human nature. This rendering of chemistry as philosophy automatically made chemistry a suitable pursuit for gentlemen of liberal education and removed chemistry from direct association with, in Adam Smith's evocative phrase, 'those only who live about the furnace'.[24] Its connotations with the craft knowledge of artisans and tradesmen were also removed. But it did not thereby remove academic chemistry from a position of acute relevance to agriculture and manufacture. With his knowledge of causative agents and specialised techniques of analysis, and insulated from the market and from the craft producer by the mediating figure of the merchant, the philosophical chemist had nonetheless a specific and significant role to play in the economic life of his community. The philosophical chemist was therefore at one and the same time the committed, improving citizen, not just because of his individual personal commitment, but by virtue of the *persona* of a philosophical chemist.

It would be hard to overstate the rhetorical brilliance and discursive adroitness of Cullen's chemistry teaching, in the way it contrived to integrate as a coherent whole the sociological, technological, philosophical and theoretorical aspects of the subject. In calling his teaching rhetoric, I do not mean to devalue his gift as merely the skilful use of words; I mean it to indicate a profoundly persuasive version of relations which did not necessarily always coincide with those that actually held outside the lecture room. We have already seen the rhetorical component of his appeal to the merchant when viewed in relation to his own situation as improver. There would indeed be other points in Cullen's chemical career where concrete situations could clash directly with Cullen's programme for chemistry and with the role of philosophical chemist-improver. At Glasgow Cullen's bold and critical promotion of an independent philosophical chemistry was made in a relatively easy situation, for medical education, and the place of chemistry within it, was not on a comparable level of either scale or systematic curriculum with that which existed in Edinburgh at mid-century. Cullen had therefore a reasonably free field in which to adapt his chemical lectureship. At Edinburgh the situation was vastly different, with chemistry having had an assigned place and role within the medical school's teaching for the past thirty years. Cullen's promotion of a chemistry independent of, among other things, the constraints of medical teaching, voiced in a public forum attended by several of the Edinburgh medical professoriate (The Edinburgh Philosophical Society) was not calculated to endear him to his future colleagues, nor further his hopes of gaining the Edinburgh chemical chair, particularly when coupled with his well-known critical attitude toward Boerhaave.[25] If this paper was an opening shot in his campaign for the Edinburgh chair, as it could plausibly be regarded, then it was deeply miscalculated, tending to trample all over the current incumbent Plummer's course, then proceeding to contradict his experimental work.[26] In another context, Cullen's role of chemist-improver was in some sense increasingly threatened, the closer he himself considered entering the market and seeking a profitable return in financial terms. There are several drafts of a letter to Lord Ilay which broached this issue with respect to salt manufacture, and the text and ensuing correspondence with Kames reveals something of an anxiety as to the consequences of such activity for how others perceived him. 'I have hitherto kept pretty clear of [the] character [of a projector]' he wrote to Lord Ilay;[27] and then when Kames told Cullen that Ilay had said he could trust his manufacturing secret with him, Cullen obviously felt slighted to be regarded as one who traded in 'secrets'.[28] Those terms, 'projector' and 'secret', were evidently redolent to Cullen of a purely commercial and self-interested approach to chemical manufacture, at odds with the self-image of the high-minded civic improver. This is only to make the straightforward point that Cullen's chemical career cannot be assumed to be automatically exemplary of the ideally typified roles and attitudes expressed in his lectures.

To counterbalance this, however, it is striking the degree to which Cullen did exemplify, in his own improving work on agriculture and bleaching, the precepts of the philosophical chemist. I have already noted Charles Withers's characterisation of Cullen's agriculture as philosophical, as being devoted to an investigation of the causal principles, above all of plant nutrition, which govern the basic processes of agriculture.[29] It is equally striking how in his chemical essay on bleaching Cullen adopted a consistently theoretical tone, and produced what amounted to a theorisation of bleaching's essential processes, in the course of which he was also developing more strictly academic research interests in the processes of evaporation and solution. One copy of this essay in the NLS Saltoun collection contains responses to Cullen's views from a practising bleacher with whom Cullen had consulted, and therefore lets one gain a sense of how the theoretical disposition of the philosophical improver and the practical knowledge of the bleacher interacted.[30] For much of the essay, the bleacher endorsed Cullen's theoretical account so far as he felt able, but more importantly, he also endorsed the practical consequences Cullen drew from his theoretical considerations. The moment of truth came however when Cullen's theory led him totally to devalue the laying out of cloth in sunlight, a process not amenable to comprehension in the terms which Cullen's theory developed. The practical bleacher at this point felt unable to acquiesce to the power of Cullen's hitherto persuasive theory. Cullen was pleased with the bleacher's responses, but even despite the caution entered by the bleacher, Cullen still betrayed some small anxiety that the bleacher's notes might be what he called 'complaisant', that is acquiescing in Cullen's opinion in order to be agreeable rather than critically honest.[31] The promotion of an independent philosophical chemistry and his applied chemical dealings with both the humble and mighty could therefore create for Cullen a series of problematic circumstances ranging from the major to the marginal.

Cullen's theoretical chemistry has so far been analysed as part of a social and educational endeavour to do with chemistry's social and academic status. It was of course considerably more than this, not simply advocacy of theory as such, but an attempt to adapt one particular and recent strand of natural philosophical theory in order to re-frame certain fundamentals of chemical understanding. This theory was one proposed by Isaac Newton as a speculative explanation for a variety of gravitational, optical, electrical, thermal and physiological effects. Newton had proposed the existence of a highly attenuated pervasive fluid, the aether, composed of extremely small corpuscles possessed of relatively powerful repelling forces.[32] Aether-based science languished throughout the 1720s and '30s in Britain, but began to revive in the 1740s.[33] Cullen called it 'the most plausible scheme of chemical philosophy',[34] and used and developed it from his early Glasgow years onward. This was a development which increasingly centralised the aether's role.[35] To begin with, Cullen had envisaged the repelling, expansive agency of aether as being counterbalanced by the micro-attractive forces of the corpuscles of ordinary matter. By the late fifties, he had abandoned the micro-forces of attraction, postulating the aether alone as universal causal agent, distributed in a field of varying densities throughout the micro-world of matter. This theory allowed Cullen to develop novel sub-sets of theories, of the states of matter, and of elective attractions, this latter being the theory most used by chemists in Britain to account for the selective or preferential nature of chemical reactivity. This research was not solely theoretical. By mid-century, the aether was increasingly identified as the material and force-substrate of both electricity and heat. Identifying the aether with the matter of heat let Cullen propose and experimentally prosecute a novel form of chemical research, a form of thermal chemistry, whereby hypothetical aether flow could be measured and quantified by detecting the thermal effect of chemical reactions. Cullen has not been regarded as any sort of quantitative chemist, partly because chemical quantification in the eighteenth century has been overwhelmingly seen as a matter of weight-relations. But what in fact Cullen pursued was an entirely novel, thermometrically quantified chemistry, in fulfilment of that Newtonian chemical dream, whereby the quantitative force relations of micro-matter could be discovered to stand alongside the macro-force quantification of gravitation which Newton had achieved. Cullen's ambitious research programme made certain strides, and he produced thermal effect tables for his students. It never however locked into place any micro-force law equivalent to universal gravitation.

That failure does not however exhaust the historical significance of Cullen's work in this field. He associated thermal effect in chemical reaction especially with solid-fluid and fluid-solid changes of state. And it was this which provided the exact and precise point of departure for his pupil Joseph Black's infinitely better known researches which discovered, conceptualised and quantified the phenomena of latent and specific heats. If it has ever appeared puzzling as to why Black, a chemist working on quick-lime and fixed air, should also and more or less simultaneously have discovered and quantified latent and specific heat, foundational physical concepts, the answer is that Cullen's research had focused Black on the relevant phenomena and had made the thermometer *par excellence* the quantifying chemist's instrument. Cullen had therefore initiated an experimental, quantifying form of investigation which was utilised for thirty years or more by his successors in the Glasgow lectureship (Black, Robison and Irvine). It was eventually passed on via Irvine's work on absolute heats, to the work of Adair Crawford in Edinburgh on animal heat. In the phenomena he sought to explain and the distinctiveness of his approach, Cullen's work therefore initiated and directed a tradition of research which came to characterise much of Scottish science in the second half of the century, and to which, moreover, the rest of his contemporary world's scientific communities could offer no precise parallel. By that is meant that whether one looks to Paris, St Petersburg, London or Philadelphia between 1750 and the 1780s, one cannot find any closely analogous case of institutionally based, quantitative experimental science, coherently devoted to one developmental sequence of topics through two generations.

Understanding the reasons for this coherence and continuity would be in a large part to understand the great strength and productivity of Scottish science in the heroic period inaugurated by Cullen. With respect to Cullen, it would be of great value if we could find out more concerning his laboratory practice than we currently know – the types and standards of instrumentation, the design of experiments, the particular procedures, techniques and skills he developed and inculcated in the young Joseph Black; such things would be very revealing if known. As yet, only a hesitant and partial start has been made on this topic, which is very difficult to investigate concretely, so I will not hazard my inadequate notions on the subject.[36]

An occasion such as this bicentenary publication is beneficial for an historian of science, because history of science is as much a field of specialised labour as any other academic area. If one were discussing progress in chemistry in the eighteenth century the contributions made by Cullen would figure in the developments which occurred in chemical theory, heat science, chemical technology, chemical education and scientific agriculture. Thus we would have (to an extent we do have) a Cullen scattered throughout specialised journals and monographs. The value of these analytical specialisms is undoubted. However, once committed to making something of a synthesis of Cullen's practice as a chemist, the divisions created by our own scholarship appear for what they are, often quite arbitrary and anachronistic. It is clear by now that Cullen was not by turns technologist, educator, philosopher, researcher; rather, with respect to chemistry, he was a committed and largely successful player of one particular role. Cullen theoretically elaborated his researches as part of his teachng, his applied chemistry was a form of theoretical work and he found it appropriate to use chemical terms such as elective attraction in discussing topics related to manure and cabbages, as well as those concerned with the higher reaches of physical theory. Given these observations the historian is surely obliged to account for this most particular form of eighteenth-century scientific life. This essay has suggested that the best way to account for such a man as Cullen is to explore what was meant by 'philosophical chemist' and what was involved in the practice of this role. In conclusion I should like to thank the Fellows, Officers and Publications Committee of the

Royal College of Physicians of Edinburgh for the opportunity to make this suggestion, and to present the finely integrated economy of Cullen's life as a chemist.

Acknowledgements

The comments of Professor Emerson and Dr Barfoot have been particularly helpful to me for rethinking certain points made in the initial version of this essay, and I take this opportunity to thank them.

Notes and references

1. A.L. Donovan, *Philosophical chemistry in the Scottish Enlightenment: the doctrines and discoveries of William Cullen and Joseph Black* (Edinburgh, 1975); J.R.R. Christie, 'The ether and the science of chemistry, 1740–90', in G.N. Cantor and M.J.S. Hodge (eds.), *Conceptions of ether: studies in ether theory, 1740–1900* (Cambridge, 1981), pp. 85–110; J.V. Golinski, *Language, method and theory in British chemical discourse, c. 1660–1770* (PhD thesis, University of Leeds, 1984), chap. E; C. Withers, 'William Cullen's agricultural lectures and writings and the development of agricultural science in eighteenth-century Scotland', *The agricultural history review*, 37 pt II (1989), pp. 144–56.
2. e.g. William Cullen, Royal College of Physicians of Edinburgh (RCPE), Cullen MSS 10.
3. *Ibid.*
4. Withers, *op cit.*
5. Aspects of this work are discussed in Donovan, *op cit.*, pp. 78–83. Cullen's work on bleaching for the Board of Trustees, of which several copies exist, elaborates on the effects of evaporation and solution for bleaching processes: Cullen 'Remarks on the Art of Bleaching or Whitening Linnen', National Library of Scotland, Saltoun Collection, MS 17569, late 1752 or early 1753.
6. Cullen's work on common salt production is discussed by Donovan, *op. cit.*, 83–6. His salt taxonomy can be found in 'Some reflections on the Study of Chemistry, and an Essay towards ascertaining the Different Species of Salts. Being part of a letter to Dr. John Clerk', read in 1753 to the Philosophical Society of Edinburgh and published in Dobbin, L., 'A Cullen chemical manuscript of 1753', *Annals of Science* 1 (1936), pp. 138–56.
7. Cullen MSS in Glasgow University Library contain lecture notes from the session 1748–9 (GUL, Cullen MSS). The library of King's College, Aberdeen has a set dated by Wightman to 1757–8 (MS Ford Y.9.3.4), and for the same session there are David Carmichael's notes in RCPE Cullen MS C 12. Sets from the 1760s are in the John Rylands Library, Manchester University (MS CH C.121), the London Medical Society (MSS 79 A–C), and RCPE (Cullen MSS 10).
8. Quoted in J. Thomson, *An account of the life, letters and writings of William Cullen, M.D.* (2 vols., vol. 1 Edinburgh 1832, vols. 1 and 2, Edinburgh, 1859), vol. 1, p. 25.
9. For Archibald Campbell in this context, see E. Cregeen, 'The changing role of the House of Argyll in the Scottish Highlands', in N.T. Phillipson and R. Mitchison (eds), *Scotland in the age of improvement*, (Edinburgh 1970) pp. 5–23; Kames conducted a voluminous scientific-improving correspondence with several men of science, and some of his improving

activities are dealt with in I.S. Ross, *Lord Kames and the Scotland of his day*, (Oxford, 1972), pp. 316–32.

10. See Withers, *op. cit.*, pp. 149–50.
11. See Cregeen, *op. cit.*, pp. 17–18.
12. Cullen, GUL Cullen MSS, 7.
13. *Ibid.*
14. E.g. Cullen, RCPE Cullen MSS 10, vol. 1, pp. 15–16.
15. Cullen, RCPE Cullen MSS 10, vol. 1, pp. 22–5.
16. For Boerhaave's 'instrumental' conception of fire, see R. Love, 'Herman Boerhaave and the element-instrument concept of fire', *Annals of Science*, 31 (1974), pp. 547–59.
17. Golinski, *op. cit.*, pp. 306–7.
18. For Shaw, Dossie and Lewis, see Golinski, *op. cit.*, chaps. D, E.
19. Cullen, RCPE, Cullen MSS 10, vol. 1, p. 26.
20. Cullen, RCPE, Cullen MSS 10, vol. 2.
21. See Golinski, *op. cit.*, chap. D, for Shaw's Baconianism.
22. Cullen, RCPE Cullen MSS 10, vol. 1, p. 26.
23. John Robison (ed.) *Lectures on the elements of chemistry, by Joseph Black, M.D.* (2 vols. Edinburgh, 1803), vol. 1, Preface, p. xxii. Robison, I think correctly, saw Cullen's transformation of chemistry as simultaneously intellectual and social.
24. A. Smith, 'The principles which lead and direct philosophical enquiries, illustrated by the history of astronomy', in J.R. Lindgren (ed.), *The early writings of Adam Smith* (New York, 1967), p. 46.
25. See Cullen, 'Some Reflections on the Study of Chemistry', in Dobbin, *op. cit.*, pp. 140–3.
26. Plummer, the occupant of the Edinburgh chair which was the focus of Cullen's chemical career ambitions, regarded Cullen as having contradicted some of his work in the 1753 paper, though whether there was any specific and technical contradiction is open to question. For Plummer's response, see Joseph Black's report to Cullen of the reception of the Cullen paper in Edinburgh: Black to Cullen in Thomson, *op. cit.*, vol. 1, pp. 58–9.
27. Cullen to Argyll, *ibid.*, p. 75.
28. Cullen to Kames, *ibid.*, p. 599.
29. Withers, *op. cit.*, p. 151.
30. Cullen, *op. cit.*, ref. 5.
31. Cullen to Kames, Thomson, *op. cit.*, pp. 76–8. I had originally thought of the bleacher's potential 'complaisance' as the deference of the practitioner to the philosophical chemist. Professor Emerson suggests however a more material reason: the bleacher had been awarded a prize by the Edinburgh Society, partly on Cullen's recommendation, and thus was indebted to Cullen. These two analyses are perhaps not incompatible, given that Cullen's power to dispose of some of the Edinburgh Society's premium funds derived in turn from his reputation as a chemist.
32. I. Newton, *Opticks* (4th ed., London, 1730). The aether speculations occur most influentially in the concluding Queries, pp. 313–82.
33. See R. Schofield, *Mechanism and materialism: British natural philosophy in the age of reason* (Princeton, 1970), chap. 4.
34. Cullen, RCPE. Cullen MSS 10, vol. 1, p. 87.
35. This point is given a more extended treatment in Christie, *op. cit.*, pp. 98–101.
36. For Cullen as a practical chemist, see J. Crellin, 'William Cullen and practical chemistry', *Actes du XIIe Congres International d'Histoire des Sciences, Paris 1968*, 6 (1971), pp. 17–21.

3

Philosophy and method in Cullen's medical teaching

MICHAEL BARFOOT

When you appeared, vain systems serv'd to blend
With endless theories the bewilder'd mind
Medicine lay bleeding with a fatal wound
And nature's self was unexplor'd around
Tho' clouds and darkness led the world astray
You rose superior, like the God of day
Dispel'd the mists that darken'd nature's face
Illum'd mankind and taught her paths to trace
Science no longer was of names the sport
Truth and truth only systems could support.[1]

But thine shall be no vulgar doom;
PHYSIC, from System's chains set free,
Now drooping sits upon thy tomb,
And mourns its Father lost in thee.[2]

In this paper I discuss some aspects of philosophy and method in William Cullen's medical teaching. Any discussion of this kind must consider how Cullen understood and used terms such as fact, theory, hypothesis and observation. However, I attempt to get away from those past and present approaches which either convict Cullen of being a 'bad' deductive theorist or defend him as a 'good' inductive observer of facts. As an alternative I offer a historical analysis of some of the pedagogical and epistemological meanings of the notion of 'system', a term which figured repeatedly in Cullen's own discussions about philosophy and method in medicine. I begin with a brief and selective review of existing commentary about Cullen's approach to medicine. I then consider some pedagogical and epistemological meanings of system in their historical context of use. Finally, I conclude with some general comments on the future directions for Cullen studies.

Cullen's commentators

All commentators on William Cullen refer to the systematic and theoretical nature of his medical work. Almost without exception, he is regarded as the last great systematiser in the eighteenth century tradition of Stahl, Hoffmann and Boerhaave.[3] Yet while this statement has been accepted as a matter of fact, judgements about the value of Cullen's particular approach have varied considerably over time. When Cullen has been referred to in recent surveys of the history of Scottish medicine, his thought is perceived as radically different from current norms in the culture of modern medicine. He discovered nothing; no new remedies were introduced by him. Many of the special functions that he attributed directly to the nervous system are now discounted. Therefore when he is described as a systematist, the term usually carries pejorative connotations, even where a commentator is quite sympathetic in other respects.[4]

Nor is this view of Cullen confined to twentieth century critics. One of the most detailed and best accounts of some aspects of Cullen's thought is in the second volume of Buckle's *History of Civilization in England* which is largely devoted to a discussion of Scotland and the 'Scotch intellect'. Buckle wrote that it must

> be deemed a remarkable proof of Cullen's love of deductive reasoning, that he, sagacious and clear sighted as he was, should have supposed that, in so practical an art as medicine, theory could, with impunity, precede practice.[5]

Buckle thought that all distinguished practising physicians had the capacity to perform rapid inductive inferences based on the detection of subtle analogies between phenomena. He argued that Cullen's 'passion for systematic and dialectic reasoning' had retarded the acquisition of such qualities.[6] Having found Cullen's practical skills wanting, Buckle went on to regard him solely as a pathologist, an area where theory was perceived to have a more legitimate and recognised role.

Buckle's empiricist and utilitarian tradition of thought was in many respects inimical to the more metaphysical approach based on first principles which characterised the eighteenth and early nineteenth century Scottish intellect. To find a quite different perspective on Cullen's achievements, it is necessary to turn to one of the patriots of that tradition, Sir William Hamilton, then professor of civil history at Edinburgh University. In his review of the first volume of John Thomson's *Life of Cullen* he wrote:

> Cullen's mind was essentially philosophic. Without neglecting observation, in which he was singularly acute, he devoted himself less to experiment than to arrangement and generalisation. We are not aware, indeed, that he made the discovery of a single sensible phenomenon.[7]

However, far from repudiating this latter point, Hamilton strongly approved. He continued:

> Nor do we think less of him that he did not. In physical science the discovery of new facts is open to every blockhead with patience, manual dexterity, and acute senses; it is less effectively promoted

by genius than by co-operation, and more frequently the result of accident than of design.[8]

Sir William used Cullen as another artillery-piece with which to bombard English intellectual culture. In this instance, however, his ammunition had already been supplied by Cullen's biographer. Thomson maintained that the systematist was also a great practitioner.[9] In an age of quackery and eponymous specifics, Cullen's so-called failure to discover or introduce any new remedies was actually regarded as an indication of his practical sagacity.[10]

Although Thomson was Cullen's first medical biographer, James Anderson, proprietor and editor of the *Bee or Weekly Literary Intelligencer*, wrote a less well-known account in 1791, the year after Cullen's death. Anderson had been taught chemistry by Cullen some thirty years beforehand and his essay was less an account of medical achievements, than an oration of feeling about Cullen the man. Anderson, like Thomson, Hamilton and Buckle later, identified the prevailing 'turn of Cullen's mind'. Instead of viewing objects individually 'as through a microscope', Cullen was presented as one who in his scientific pursuits

> takes a sweeping view of the universe at large, considers every object he perceives, not individually, but as part of one harmonious whole: his mind is, therefore, not so much employed in examining the separate parts of this individual object, as in tracing its relations, connection, and dependencies on those around it.[11]

However, he also pointed out that Cullen's talent was not restricted to 'arrangement' alone: he was equally distinguished by his ability to separate true from false facts, which then constituted the raw materials for subsequent generalisations.

This brief survey of opinions shows that the views of the Englishman Buckle differ from those put forward by Cullen's Scottish commentators, Anderson, Thomson and Hamilton. Whereas they all acknowledged the systematic, theoretical, and relational form of Cullen's thinking, Buckle used this as an explanation of Cullen's failure to discover any medical facts and his apparent lack of reputation as a practising physician. The Scots disagreed. They argued that Cullen's doctrines, in another aspect, could be seen as a series of general facts which had been arrived at inductively by an enumeration of other facts of a less general nature. The implication was that Cullen in his dual role as teacher and practitioner of medicine relied upon the same underlying powers of accurate observation.[12]

Both these responses to Cullen have their origin in the tide of inductivism which swept nineteenth century British medicine and science It is also clear that our own preoccupation with a similar set of problems has to a large extent inhibited the historical understanding of Cullen's system in its original context of use.

Historians of medicine, asked today what Cullen's system consisted of, might well say it was the sum total of his views on medicine, and how they were related to one another through an overall emphasis upon the nervous system.[13] This is understandable. With the hindsight provided by his unpublished lecture notes and papers, as well as the published works, it is indeed tempting to equate Cullen's system with the content of his medical discourse as a whole. Yet the possibility of treating Cullen's system as the totality of his discourse only arose as a result of Thomson's dual activities as Cullen's editor and biographer.[14] As well as identifying the extent of Cullen studies, Thomson also directed the subsequent course of scholarship towards the problem of nervous action. Treating Cullen's system as virtually coterminous with his view of the nervous system has come to predominate because it gives us exactly what it gave Thomson: a way of unifying the various contents of Cullen's discourse.

Once again, this account of Cullen's system would not correspond to the various historical meanings it had in its original context of use. For example, it is not what the majority of Cullen's eighteenth century students usually understood as his system of medicine, although it may well have been part of it. Their view, the view from below as it were, was far less coherent in terms of a unifying content than our own. This is because their education intersected with Cullen's professorial career in a variety of different ways. This incompatibility between the historical meaning of system and its reconstruction as the totality of his discourse can be made most forcefully by reviewing Cullen's teaching career, and then putting oneself in the position of an eighteenth-century Edinburgh medical student best placed to hear and read about his views.

Cullen's system as pedagogy

Cullen taught for over forty years. His career stretched from his first appearance as an extramural medical teacher at Glasgow in 1744–5, to shortly before his death, when he began but was unable to complete the November 1789–May 1790 session. The combinations of different subjects he lectured upon during this period are displayed in the diagram on p. 115, along with the dates of his publications and professorial appointments.[15] A student who attended for more than one session between 1769–70 and 1773–4 would have had the benefit of successive courses on the theory and practice of physic as a result of the arrangement with John Gregory whereby each professor lectured alternately on both subjects.[16] He would also have had an opportunity of attending Cullen's clinical lectures in the Infirmary.[17] If he studied after 1769, he could supplement his course work with the *Nosology*; if after 1772, with the *Physiology*.[18] He could also get some idea of Cullen's views on the materia medica in the pirated *Lectures on the Materia Medica* of 1772.[19] However, that same student would still be subject to the vicissitudes of Cullen's digressive mode of lecturing with infrequent reference to short notes only, which often resulted in significant sections of each course being omitted. Unless he was prepared to repeat the institutes or theory of medicine lectures at least once, possibly twice, he would almost certainly be deficient in at least some parts of physiology, pathology and therapeutics.[20] Nor at this time would he have had the benefit of the *First Lines of the Practice of Physic* to complement and, more especially, to guide his study of parts of the practice course omitted for similar reasons.[21] Also, the same student would lack the benefits of Cullen's final say on materia medica and therapeutics in the *Treatise* of 1789.[22] The deficiencies experienced by other students attending either before 1769 or after 1775 were even more glaring, especially after the latter date when Cullen gave up clinical lecturing as well as the institutes of medicine.[23] Therefore what the students understood and referred to as Cullen's 'system' was not, and indeed could not have been, equivalent to the totality of his medical doctrines found in lectures and publications.

Instead of thinking of Cullen's system as a totality of discourse, the students were more familiar with another meaning of 'system' which Cullen inculcated in the classroom. 'System' in this most basic sense referred simply to an organised body of opinions on particular topics in the medical curriculum. For example, he might offer a 'short system of sympathy'; on another occasion he even referred to his 'system' of mercury treatment.[24] It would also have made perfect sense for Cullen to have referred to his system of the nervous system although, for obvious reasons, he tended to substitute 'theory' for 'system' in this particular instance. When Cullen began his first complete course of the theory and practice of physic he spoke of giving 'an entire System of Medicine'.[25] After 1777, when he referred to his 'system', on some occasions he meant all the doctrines contained in the *First Lines* or some part of them such as the role of spasm in fevers. Thus 'system', although it implied subject matter of some kind, also referred to the way in which the contents were organised and presented in a general or theoretical way. Hence Benjamin Rush commented that Cullen 'had a great Turn for System, [and] arranged all his Lectures in such a manner that it was hard to tell [whether] most to admire their Ingenuity or their Order'.[26]

The utility of acquiring medical knowledge by system for the medical students becomes apparent from a consideration of well-known features of the eighteenth century medical curriculum at Edinburgh University. Cullen's classes were part of a much wider range of courses which were

CULLEN'S TEACHING CAREER

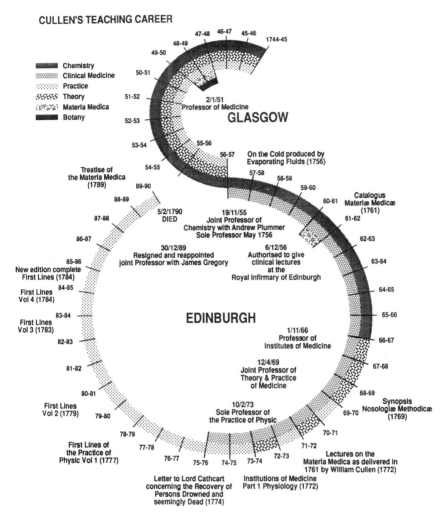

Chemistry
Clinical Medicine
Practice
Theory
Materia Medica
Botany

1744-45
47-48 46-47 45-46
48-49
49-50
50-51
51-52
52-53
53-54
54-55
55-56
56-57 On the Cold produced by Evaporating Fluids (1756)
57-58
58-59
59-60

2/1/51 Professor of Medicine
GLASGOW

Treatise of the Materia Medica (1789)
89-90
88-89
87-88
86-87
85-86 New edition complete First Lines (1784)

First Lines Vol 4 (1784) 84-85
First Lines Vol 3 (1783) 83-84
82-83
81-82
80-81
First Lines Vol 2 (1779) 79-80
78-79
First Lines of the Practice of Physic Vol 1 (1777) 77-78
76-77 75-76 74-75 73-74 72-73

5/2/1790 DIED
19/11/55 Joint Professor of Chemistry with Andrew Plummer Sole Professor May 1756
30/12/89 Resigned and reappointed joint Professor with James Gregory

6/12/56 Authorised to give clinical lectures at the Royal Infirmary of Edinburgh

EDINBURGH

1/11/66 Professor of Institutes of Medicine

12/4/69 Joint Professor of Theory & Practice of Medicine

10/2/73 Sole Professor of the Practice of Physic

Letter to Lord Cathcart concerning the Recovery of Persons Drowned and seemingly Dead (1774)
Institutions of Medicine Part 1 Physiology (1772)
Lectures on the Materia Medica as delivered in 1761 by William Cullen (1772)

71-72
70-71
69-70 Synopsis Nosologiæ Methodicæ (1769)
68-69
67-68
66-67
65-66
64-65
63-64
62-63
61-62
60-61 Catalogus Materiæ Medicæ (1761)

taught by different professors at different times. The *laissez-faire* organisation of the University during this period has been discussed by Morrell.[27] The competition for fees among professors, the relationship between pedagogy and practice, and the highly individualistic character of medical culture at this time, all encouraged the development of rival and conflicting medical opinions.[28] Divergences between some of Cullen's views and those of other University professors were pointed out by the followers of John Brown, Cullen's ex-pupil and extramural rival.[29] Even professors such as James Gregory acknowledged as much.[30] From the student's viewpoint, the various branches of an

Edinburgh medical education then available corresponded less to a carefully cultivated Georgian landscaped garden and more to an overgrown plantation.[31] The conflicting accounts of the animal economy which students received as they moved from classroom to classroom should not be underestimated.[32] Faced with this eclectic and confusing situation, the pragmatic adoption of a particular professor's system had much to commend it.

This argument about the utility of learning by system can be pushed further. It could be argued that, for students, the validity of Cullen's opinions was not at issue; it was the coherence that mattered. To ascribe uncompromisingly instrumentalist attitudes to the students, however, would be to discount what we already know about their motivation from diaries and correspondence.[33] Although some students probably adopted a cynical attitude to their studies, the vast majority believed they were there to acquire the necessary knowledge to care for the sick in the best way possible.[34] Some were even inspired by the prospect of improving medicine, should it fall to their lot to do so. The content, truth and value of medical knowledge also mattered to them, and this is very apparent in the sincerity of the debates about Cullen's ideas.[35] Ironically, it is not the attitudes of the attending students, but rather the grounds upon which Cullen commended his own system that presents a problem.

Although Cullen was active as a consulting physician[36] and made an interesting foray into the arena of medical police or public health,[37] most of his medical discourse was produced in conjunction with his role as an educator of young physicians.[38] He explicitly drew attention to the psychological advantages of adopting a system as an integral part of the process of learning medicine; it gave 'order [and] coherence [and] therefore more ready apprehension [and] more easy recollections'.[39] Nor were the advantages of system restricted to the student in the classroom but applied equally to a newly-qualified practitioner faced with his first real patient. For example, he advised a former pupil, Dr Balfour Russell, to devote time to

> perfecting yourself in some system. Few people but professors do so; but everyone that would appear in the learned world ought to do it. The system may be what you please; but I would prefer the Practice of Physic as connected with your daily employment; . . . You will not find it possible to separate practice from theory altogether; and therefore if you have a mind to begin with the theory, I have no objection.[40]

Cullen's apparent attitude here certainly gave Buckle cause for concern and, in fact, the precise grounds upon which Cullen commended his system itself became a matter of public debate ten years after his death. James Gregory, professor of the theory of medicine and Cullen's eventual successor to the senior chair, clearly thought that Cullen's justification for teaching and learning by system was purely psychological. In his *Memorial to the Managers of the Royal Infirmary* he recounted a conversation about the propriety of delivering a system of medicine to students which he said had passed between Cullen and his father, John Gregory:

> 'There must be a Tub to amuse the Whale,' said DR CULLEN to my father, who had expressed his concern at seeing so many of our students mis-spend their time and labour in that manner, and had even taken the liberty of a friend and colleague to remonstrate a little with him on some of his own favourite speculations, neither the truth nor the usefulness of which my father could perceive.[41]

He explained that Cullen sought to create a psychological condition in the minds of his listeners which James Gregory described as 'ardour in the pursuits of science'. Even if this was 'ill-directed' and 'wasted on frivolous subjects', Cullen believed that without it, no one would ever make progress in medicine.[42] Gregory considered Cullen's system was largely compiled out of false hypotheses and theories, and therefore it was actually misleading for students. As an austere, common sense Aberdonian, taught to applaud the virtues of sober and chaste induction, Gregory questioned the value of 'ardour' in medicine and was inclined to associate it with 'enthusiasm' and even 'phrenzy'.

In his *Answer* to Gregory, John Bell criticised these remarks because they implied a certain want of sincerity and even cynicism on Cullen's part and were inconsistent with his public standing as an educator of young physicians.[43] In the *Additional Memorial* Gregory sought to temper his comments as follows:

> [Cullen's] meaning plainly was, that while he endeavoured to instruct his pupils in the well established and useful facts and principles of physic, which are often dry and tedious, sometimes even disgusting, it was necessary to beguile and animate them on their weary way, by amusing them with more pleasing prospects, and engaging them in pursuits, which, by rousing them to active exertions, might quicken progress in their toilsome journey; even while they seemed to withdraw them farthest from the common beaten track.[44]

From this passage, it is apparent that Gregory allowed Cullen had on occasions provided his students with useful facts in the practice of medicine.[45] Yet because they were transmitted in conjunction with the theoretical and hypothetical parts of Cullen's system, he continued to question the balance between entertainment and real instruction in Cullen's teaching, especially of the institutes.[46]

It is clear that Gregory's statement of the relationship between facts and theory in Cullen's system differs from Anderson, Hamilton and Thomson and is closer to, although not identical with, Buckle's. In

principle, Gregory seems to have allowed there was a legitimate role for
system considered as general theory or some kind of a connecting
medium which linked facts together. Nevertheless he distinguished
between this and the kind of theorising or system-building which Cullen
had indulged in.[47] Once again, the relationship between medical theory
and facts seems to be at the heart of understanding Cullen's systematic
approach to medicine. Therefore it seems appropriate to look in more
detail at Cullen's epistemological views on the need for system and the
various roles he accorded to theory, observation, hypothesis and fact in
relation to it.

Cullen's system as epistemology

The principal published source for Cullen's remarks on system is the
'Lectures introductory to the course on the practice of physic', included
by Thomson in his edition of the *Works*. Thomson used 'copies
corrected in Dr Cullen's hand-writing' to compile the text, which is
subdivided into sections on history of medicine, method of study, plan
of course, and on nosology.[48] Cullen's sense of teaching and learning by
medical system was thoroughly historical. He gave an account of the
development of medicine to students commencing the practice of physic
course, much as he had done for chemistry earlier.[49] Cullen claimed to
'deduce the history of physic through many ages' and he clearly
conceived of his narrative as a contribution to the 'literary history of
physic'. Despite the reliance on written sources, it was similar in form to
conjectural or theoretical history, much loved by the Scots in general.[50]
Gaps in the historical record and deficiencies of testimony were filled by
imaginative reasoning, and this gave ample scope for generalisation and
speculative disquisition. In the hands of exponents such as Lord Kames,
Adam Smith and David Hume, the genre was mainly concerned with
the rise and progress of society. However, the institutionalisation of
human knowledge was also frequently discussed as one very important
aspect of social change. Philosophical histories of particular disciplines,
considered within the framework of the rise and progress of the arts and
sciences, also became something of a specialty of some Scottish
professors.[51]

Working within this broad tradition, Cullen presented a history of
what might

> be called the Revolutions of physic – that is an account of the
> changes which, from time to time, have happened in the method of
> cultivating the art, with the general effects of these as well as
> history will allow us to discern them.[52]

He classified the history of medicine into seven periods. However, the
actual divisions are less important than the mechanisms of change
Cullen identified in the revolutions from one period to another. Period

one was characterised as a 'natural state of physic' in which medical practice first arose from a combination of instinct, spontaneous cures, accidental errors and random trials. The earliest practitioners relied on observation and experience alone, and therefore conducted themselves on the empiric plan. The first revolution occurred when society slowly became more refined and this, in turn, led to the cultivation of theory. This gave rise to a second period in which medicine was practised on the dogmatic plan. It coincided with the rise of the ancient schools, stretching from 400–287 BC, and Cullen called it the period of ancient dogmatism.

With the exception of a period of formal empiricism which succeeded ancient dogmatism,[53] Cullen argued that all the other revolutions in the practice of medicine had followed from innovations in theory. He wrote that it was only 'the combination of philosophy with a knowledge of the facts of physic, that could make any considerable change in the state of the art.'[54] Change, then, was dependent upon the state of refinement in society and, in particular, on the prevailing 'ardour in the culture of philosophy'. Whenever literature and the arts were cultivated or neglected, medicine became a mirror of the wider situation. Although Cullen marked the periods and revolutions of medicine by the historical figures prominently associated with new approaches, the emphasis was very much on those conditions promoting change which had a much broader basis than the actions of great men. As he succinctly put it: 'no man can go much further than the state of science at his particular period allows him.'[55]

While Cullen linked the fate of medicine with 'the general culture of the human mind', its progress was also dependent upon additional conditions being fulfilled. Like forms of natural knowledge in general, medicine relied upon experience which

> can only be acquired by many hands and repeated labours; it can only be the uninterrupted work of many ages, secured in leisure, provided with proper instruments, and admitted to a communication with all the parts of the globe.[56]

Cullen did not enter into the prevailing social conditions which had recently set medicine on the road to improvement, other than to characterise the seventh and final era of physic as 'an inquisitive and industrious age'. However, his descriptions of the period from the discovery of the circulation of the blood to Boerhaave implied that such conditions were increasingly being met in his own lifetime.

As well as necessary changes in the social milieu, Cullen identified the methodological and intellectual landmarks of the modern period which had also guided progress. Methodologically, the innovations of Galileo and Bacon deeply affected the kind of dogmatism which prevailed in his time. Mechanical philosophers were largely responsible for fashioning modern dogmatism, and this was distinct from other kinds because its advocates had not neglected observation and experiment while pursuing theory and hypotheses. Not only had this redeeming quality enabled them to detect the falsity of previous hypotheses, it also

> established the innocence of the theories of the present age, that the particular inferences drawn from them are always subjected to the test of experience; and with regard to the most noted leaders in them . . . it can hardly be alleged that their speculations have ever slackened their diligence in observation and experiment, or rendered them adverse to those presented by others.[57]

Intellectually, Cullen regarded the discoveries of the circulation of the blood and the course of the chyle as the crucial developments, because they gave 'the proper view of the hydraulic apparatus in the animal economy.'[58] Once these intellectual discoveries were firmly in place, physicians were finally in a position to attempt systems of medicine. When

> many new facts have been acquired, it becomes requisite that these should be incorporated into a system, whereby not only particular subjects may be improved, but the whole may be rendered more complete, consistent, and useful. Every system, indeed, must be valuable in proportion to the number of facts that it embraces and comprehends . . .[59]

Such facts had led to views of the animal economy as an 'hydraulic machine', as well as a 'chemical mixt'. Recent discoveries about the nervous system promised to add the further dimension of an 'animated nervous frame'.[60]

Whereas earlier, Cullen had emphasised the pivotal role of theory in producing those general revolutions in medicine which had occurred historically, facts acquired greater importance as a driving force of change in the progressive contemporary period of physic. Therefore when he discussed the role of facts in the period of modern dogmatism, many of his statements do not appear dramatically different from the standard eighteenth-century position. Progress was often interpreted in terms of the gradual collection and accumulation of facts in order to arrive at general laws or first principles by induction. However, Cullen's conception of what a fact actually consisted of was strikingly different from the majority of his contemporaries. He stated that we

> do and must assume that the facts of physic are more frequently the inferences of reason than the simple objects of sense, and therefore that the bringing out of the facts that are necessary, and the ascertaining them to be such, will always proceed in proportion to our advances in the knowledge of system, and that truly an empiric system can hardly be perfect till the dogmatic is nearly so.[61]

Cullen was distinctive, possibly even alone, in rejecting the theory-free conception of facts in medicine which was part and parcel of the orthodox view.[62] In the introductory lectures, as well as elsewhere in his writings, he argued forcefully that a medical fact was the product of theoretical reasoning, and that its usefulness depended upon its wider role within a particular system of medicine. He explained the growth of medical knowledge in terms of an interaction between established facts and new theories and which took place within systems, guided by the methodology of the mechanical dogmatism of the seventh period of physic. He wrote that in studying the dogmatic plan

> we must often try hypotheses. I hold the practice safe and useful; safe if it is only employed for leading to facts and experiments, and highly useful if it does so. Hypotheses have been much decried, and justly, because they have been abused; but, at the same time, I am persuaded that they are almost unavoidable, and have been more useful than is commonly believed; for they have often produced facts that would otherwise have passed unheeded, and experiments that would otherwise not have been made.[63]

Cullen's lectures on the history of medicine charted the rise of modern dogmatism and drew attention to the important role it had played in both the genesis of medical facts and the formulation of systems put forward by Stahl, Hoffman and Boerhaave. However, Cullen did not only preach the principles of dogmatic medicine in the classroom; he also put them into effect in the clinical setting. In this context, a hitherto unmentioned aspect of modern dogmatism emerges most clearly – its philosophical scepticism with regard to matters of fact.

His clinical lectures of 1772–3 presented Cullen's students with a bleak picture of the limited progress hitherto made in compiling factual case histories of particular diseases.

> From Novelty, Omission, Mistake, design &c. our medical Histories are necessarily incomplete, erroneous and false, and so not at all sufficient to enable us to distinguish diseases from one another and are unfit for founding a decisive practice.[64]

Without a clear understanding of the facts of disease, Cullen argued, it was impossible to arrive at 'Methodical Nosology', or the classification of diseases into species by an enumeration of their pathognomic symptoms.[65] By the same token, imperfections in nosological classification further hindered the discovery and distinction of medical facts:

> Everybody will find it necessary to attempt a System of Nosology and unless he is attempting to refer his facts to such a System he will overlook and mistake facts . . . however imperfect that State of our Science may be, it does not hinder us to refer facts to it in order to digest and correct them.[66]

Cullen's view of the relationship between nosological theory and the facts of case histories is a further example of the dialectical relationship between theory and fact in general found throughout his writings. However, there is also a noticeable difference of emphasis in the clinical lectures. The institutes and history of medicine lectures reveal Cullen's overall tendency to justify the role of theory. In the clinical lectures, greater stress is placed upon the need to acquire accurate facts about the distinction of disease and the operation of remedies. When he descended to the details of particular cases, Cullen was prepared to share his own doubts about the 'facts' of disease. His discourse in the clinical setting is characterised by hesitations, apologies, revisions and admission of mistakes. He claimed it was a conscious decision to reveal his practice in this way and that he could have hidden many of his errors by subterfuge. However, he believed that error was as instructive as apparent success. In doing so, Cullen was consciously playing out the role of the sceptical dogmatist.

In the final lecture, he gave an account of the general causes leading to the 'uncertainty and fallacy that subsist with regard to distinguishing disease' in the belief that it would help 'direct to the means of remedying them'.[67] Adopting the motto that 'fore warned is half armed', Cullen encouraged his students to be suspicious of any case reports which displayed the following characteristics: having few or incomplete details; containing superstitious or credulous testimony; and revealing a bias towards system and a partiality for particular remedies. All these shortcomings were attributed to the fallacies of sense, the weaknesses of human understanding and the passions and interests of men.

It is important to note that, despite his scepticism, Cullen did not deny the existence of medical facts as such. He commented:

> I hope true facts there are, and if we have endeavoured to collect these under the correction of doubts and suspicions that I have just now mentioned, that we are only able to judge what is probable and possible w[it]h reg[ar]d to the human body.[68]

However, he reiterated the fundamental point that true facts were not to be acquired independently of analogical reasoning but by means of it, and that all the accepted facts in physic were the results of some kind of reasoning. Empiric medicine was fallacious, if not impossible, because 'every person who has attempted to give a system of practice founded upon facts . . . is running every moment into System, and is commonly only endeavouring to form a rope of sand.'[69] Because reasoning was a form of theory and theory of some kind was inevitable, it followed that some form of dogmatism – albeit an unconscious one – was also unavoidable.

Cullen appears to have liked the image of a rope of sand as he also used it in his institutes course, this time in a much broader context.

> In short, the whole of human Life, Society, [and] the Actions of all men are determined by this Law of Habit. Many men are engaged

in a certain Rotine [*sic*] of Actions, which they cannot be withdrawn from. Society, without these Associations from Habit would be as (what we would say) a rope of Sand, without any connection together.[70]

At this precise point, Cullen was actually discussing habitual actions performed by the body. Yet it is clear that he adopted an identical perspective when it came to the association of ideas 'which is the foundation of memory and all our intellectual faculties, and is entirely the effect of custom; its influence on morals is very great . . .'.[71] For Cullen, system was unavoidable not simply because of man's love of theorising, but because it necessarily reflected the way the mind worked. His whole approach to medicine was framed in relation to a particular metaphysic of mind which he shared – in outline at least – with Hume, Smith, and Hutton among his Scottish contemporaries, and Hartley and Priestley in England.[72] This is seen at work most clearly in his account of causality.

Cullen conceded that, in nature, causes and effects were connected in a circle and therefore, in some sense, everything was related to everything else.[73] However medicine, like all other forms of natural knowledge, best proceeded by connecting phenomena in terms of causal chains composed of customary constant conjunctions of antecedents and consequents.[74] An identical approach can be found in his insistence that, from a medical point of view, the relation between body and mind must be treated as if it were one of physical necessity. If mind was allowed to act arbitrarily in relation to the body then, Cullen argued, it would be impossible for us to reason or even speak meaningfully about medical matters.

Cullen's system therefore was not mechanical in the sense that he always allowed a pervasive role for the operation of mind upon the body. Rather he appears to have conceded that, on occasions, the mind might act upon the body in ways that were not traceable physically. Yet he maintained that there was no choice but to infer the action of the mind by its effects on the body.[75] Thus the form of reasoning he employed while discussing the animal economy was necessarily mechanical and, in this respect, he sometimes referred to it as 'the mechanic reasoning', and this is the meaning he sought to convey when he characterised the seventh period of physic as an era of mechanical dogmatism.[76] It is this necessitarian theory of causal judgement, applied to the animal economy generally and the nervous system in particular, which distinguishes Cullen's medical thought from his voluntarist contemporaries.[77] Considered as a product of association, his system was a necessarily determined network of relations of ideas held together by the customary transition of the imagination and nothing else. Yet for all that, Cullen remained a sceptical dogmatist rather than an out-and-out sceptic as such. His use of scepticism in the classroom and at the bedside was always of the mitigated and not Pyrrhonian kind, which he viewed as an 'exercise of wit' which had 'no influence on human conduct'.

> Suppose me in my easy chair this morning ruminating on the doctrines of Sceptics [and] plunged into absolute doubt about every thing[.] My wife comes in [and] minds me it is time to dress [and] go to the College[.] I consider whether I shall go or not. Many Arguments offer[.] My Engagements are strong both in honour [and] interest[.] [T]hese presently set me dressing.[78]

Conclusion

Approaching questions of philosophy and method in Cullen's discourse through an analysis of the historical meanings of system has much to commend it. Instead of turning into a formal exercise in the philosophy of method, judged by current understandings, it is possible to appreciate the variety of levels, institutional, pedagogical, psychological and epistemological, upon which Cullen's system operated. I have placed the greatest emphasis upon three interrelated sets of meanings. First, system implied a psychological pedagogy within a specific institutional setting. Secondly, it embodied a methodological stance towards theory, observation and the role of hypotheses within observational and experimental practice. And thirdly it encouraged an attitude of philosophical scepticism with regard to matters of fact.

For narrative convenience the discussion began with a consideration of the pedagogical uses of Cullen's system before proceeding to consider its epistemological meanings. However, this is an artificial segregation. When he spoke as a philosopher of medicine, Cullen was also fulfilling his role as a university professor. System was simultaneously an expression of the necessary order of the human mind and a pedagogical strategy. It is also important to note that it was very much a part of Cullen's argument that for sceptical dogmatism to be of real value, it also had to embrace the practice as well as the theory of physic. System had to guide action at the bedside, and not just serve as a means of organising medical knowledge in the classroom.

As the aim throughout is to draw attention to Cullen's philosophical attitude to medicine, little attention has been paid to topics such as health and disease, nervous ether and spasm, sensibility and irritability, custom and passion, excitement and collapse and the notions of periodicity and fitness, all of which are important for understanding the details of Cullen's approach to the animal economy. Ultimately, Cullen's philosophy of method cannot be separated from the contents of his particular medical doctrines. Nevertheless, there are advantages to be gained by segregating them in this somewhat artificial way. Some original and hitherto unacknowledged aspects of Cullen's method are highlighted and the general analysis of his system of medicine helps us to understand and explain the specific doctrines he held about the animal economy. A greater understanding of Cullen's pervasive attitude to the possibility of progressive medical knowledge, of how it should be acquired and of the necessary form it should take prepares the way for a more detailed account of Cullen's views in a manner which does not reduce everything to different aspects of the nervous system. This will make Cullen a less consistent medical writer, but ultimately a more interesting one.

Finally, the multiple historical roles played by Cullen's system help us to understand why his eighteenth and nineteenth century commentators emphasised different aspects of his discourse. By selective interpretation, it was easy to construe him as a deductive theorist or as a cautious seeker of medical facts. Commentators in the twentieth century, however, have fewer excuses for treating Cullen in this manner. It is certainly possible to find rhetorical statements by Cullen about the inductive method which commend it in that general and unreflective manner which is characteristic of so much eighteenth century discourse. At the same time, Cullen did offer substantive analyses of the nature of a fact and its relationship to theory. Therefore a more careful reading of the Cullen archives offers great scope for seeing him as a medical thinker whose conception of philosophical method in medicine was immeasurably more sophisticated than the consensus of his day. In many respects, it is closer to explanations favoured by those present-day philosophers, sociologists and historians whose explanations of scientific and medical change have acknowledged the complexity of the interaction which takes place between theory and data. However, Cullen's sophistication is not just due to his philosophical acumen, although it is clear that like so many of his Scottish contemporaries, he was remarkably well-informed about metaphysics. He also sought an understanding of medicine in terms of its historical development within society. For Cullen, the facts of medicine endorsed by contemporary dogmatists were as much the products of history as the theories of Galen or Boerhaave. It is this consciousness of the historical process which holds out the most promise for establishing a common philosophical outlook between Cullen and his friends and sometime patients, Hume and Smith.

Acknowledgements

Thanks go to staff at Special Collections, Glasgow University Library, the National Library of Scotland, the Library of the Royal College of Physicians, and to my colleagues at Special Collections, Edinburgh University Library for their assistance and for permission to quote from manuscript material. I am grateful to Lothian Health Board and the

Royal Infirmary of Edinburgh for their support of the Medical Archive Centre.

Notes and references

Abbreviations: EUL, Edinburgh University Library; GUL, Glasgow University Library; NLS, National Library of Scotland; RCPE, Library of the Royal College of Physicians of Edinburgh. All quotations from manuscript material are in Cullen's hand unless otherwise identified as a transcription.

1. Untitled poem by unknown author in 'Letters to Dr Cullen'. 3 vols, RCPE Cullen MS 32. vol. 1, 1790 (unpaginated).
2. Armstrong, J., 'Verses on the death of Dr Cullen'. In Cullen, ref. 1, vol. 1 (unpaginated).
3. The location of Cullen within the great tradition of medical systematists has its origins in Thomson, J., *An account of the life, lectures and writings of William Cullen, M.D.* 2 vols., Edinburgh: Blackwood, 1859, vol. 1 (originally published 1832): 162–258.
4. For example see Hamilton, D., *The healers: a history of medicine in Scotland*, Edinburgh: Canongate, 1981: 135: 'Cullen is not associated with any major research discovery nor did he promote any lasting insight into disease or therapy.' See also Comrie, J.D., *History of Scottish medicine*, 2 vols., London: Wellcome Historical Medical Museum, 1932, vol. 1: 314: 'In [Cullen's] day, theories as to the nature of life and vital processes were considered all-important, a matter which is difficult to understand in the present age, when the human mind accepts the mystery of life as a fact, and inquires only into the ways in which it is manifested.'
5. Buckle, H.T., *History of civilization in England*, 2nd edn. 2 vols., London: Parker, 1861, vol. 2: 537–8.
6. *Ibid.*, 538.
7. [Hamilton, W.] Review of 'Life of Cullen', *Edin. Rev.* 1832: 55: 461. These remarks were reiterated in Garrison, F.H., *An introduction to the history of medicine*, 4th ed. Philadelphia and London: Saunders, 1929: 358: 'Sir William Hamilton was perilously near the truth when he said that "Cullen did not add a single new fact to medical science."'
8. Hamilton, ref. 7: 461.
9. Thomson, ref. 3, vol. 1: 107–21.
10. Anon. Death of Dr John Thomson, *Scotsman*, 17 October 1846: 'in the character of a prescribing physician, he ever aimed at simplicity . . . it was a favourite expression of his, that . . . Dr Cullen [had never] introduced a new remedy.'
11. [Anderson, J.] Cursory hints and anecdotes of the late Doctor William Cullen of Edinburgh, *The Bee, or literary weekly intelligencer* 1790–1; *1*: 122.
12. See Thomson, ref. 3, vol. 2: 94–8; Hamilton, ref. 7: 239: Anderson, ref. 11: 123–4. The present-day successor to what might be called the Scottish patriot tradition of reading Cullen is George Davie. See his *The democratic intellect: Scotland and her universities in the nineteenth century*, Edinburgh: Edinburgh University Press, 1962: 23: 'There was in the Faculty of Medicine, too, an analogous tendency to keep alive questions of first principle as a guide to research and practice. The seminal mind here, probably , was that of Cullen . . . [who sought to find] a general theory of disease which would connect up with speculation about the nature of life and its relations to mind and matter.'
13. See Bowman, I.A., *William Cullen (1710–90) and the primacy of the nervous system*, Indiana University: PhD thesis, 1975; Lawrence, C.J.,

Medicine as culture: Edinburgh and the Scottish Enlightenment, University College London: PhD thesis, 1984: 312–416.

14. Cullen, W., *The works of William Cullen, M.D. . . . containing his physiology, nosology, and first lines of the practice of physic: with numerous extracts from his manuscript papers, and from his treatise of the materia medica*. Ed. Thomson, J., 2 vols., Edinburgh: Blackwood, 1827.

15. The diagram refers to winter sessions of lectures only which stretched from November to April or May. The distribution of courses in Glasgow is based on information contained in Thomson's *Life* and should be treated cautiously. The Edinburgh courses can be checked against other sources and are more reliably ascertained. For the sake of simplicity, Cullen's various summer and extramural courses have not been included.

16. Some of the best student transcriptions of Cullen's institutes lectures come from this period. For example, see 'Lectures on the institutions of medicine by Dr Cullen, 1771–2', NLS MS 3535. It has recently been suggested that this is in Cullen's hand and can therefore serve as a preferred text for understanding Cullen's views. See Wright, J.P., 'Metaphysics and physiology: mind, body and the animal economy in eighteenth-century Scotland', In Stewart, M.A., (ed.) *Studies in the philosophy of the Scottish Enlightenment*, Oxford: Clarendon, 1990: 251. It is worth emphasising that Cullen always lectured from notes only, and where we do have lectures written in his own hand they are in note form. There are essays on specific doctrines such as fever, the vis medicatrix naturae, health, hypochondria, custom and the history of medicine (see ref. 38). However, the fully written-out lecture notes are either student copies, or transcriptions of an amanuensis, some of which have been corrected in Cullen's distinctive hand. Therefore it is very unlikely that there are any complete transcriptions of Cullen's lectures solely in his own hand which could serve as a preferred text.

17. See, for example, Cullen, W., 'Clinical lectures 1772–3', 4 vols, RCPE MS 4. Apart from Cullen's increasing popularity, another reason for the completeness of lecture notes at this time was the appearance of new and popular short-hand primers. See Byrom, J., *The universal English short-hand*, Manchester: Harrop. 1767; Holdsworth, W., and Aldridge, W., *Natural short-hand system*, London: Wells and Grosvenor, [1768].

18. [Cullen, W.] *Synopsis nosologiae methodicae*, Edinburgh: (no publisher) 1769; [Cullen, W.] *Institutions of medicine. Part 1. Physiology*. For the use of the students in the University of Edinburgh, Edinburgh: (no publisher) 1772.

19. See [Cullen, W.] *Lectures on the materia medica, as delivered by William Cullen . . . and now printed from a correct copy, which has been compared with others by the editors*. London: T. Lowndes, 1772. A corrected edition was published with Cullen's consent in the following year.

20. See, for example, Cullen, ref. 16: 354–77, where the discussion of pathology was restricted to the nervous system only.

21. Cullen, W., *First lines of the practice of physic for the use of students in the University of Edinburgh*, 4 vols., Edinburgh and London: Murray, Creech, Elliot, and Cadell 1777–1784. (Vol. 2, 1779; vol. 3, 1783; vol. 4, 1784.) A number of editions and impressions appeared. The student who transcribed MS 3535 (ref. 16) may well have gone on to transcribe 'Cullen's Practice'. NLS MSS 3536–3537 in the following session. However, it is noticeable that these lectures are far less complete than other copies written after vol. 1 of the *First lines* appeared.

22. Cullen, W., *A treatise of the materia medica*, 2 vols., Edinburgh: Elliot and Kay, 1789.

23. The only published details of Cullen's clinical teaching appeared seven

years after his death. See *Clinical lectures, delivered in the years 1765 and 1766, by William Cullen, M.D. . . . taken in short-hand by a gentleman who attended*, London: Lee and Hurst, 1797.

24. See Cullen, ref. 16: 199; and ref. 17, vol. 3: 632.

25. Cullen, W., 'Lectures on physiology', 5 vols., RCPE MS 18, vol. 1: 1.

26. Rush, B., 'Journal, 1766–68', EUL Mic M 28: 60.

27. Morrell, J.B., 'The University of Edinburgh in the 18th century: its scientific eminence and academic structure', *Isis* 1971; *62*: 158–71.

28. Morrell, J.B., 'Individualism and the structure of British science in 1830', *Hist. Stud. Phys. Sci.* 1971; *3*: 183–204. Although this article describes scientific culture generally for a somewhat later period, it applies equally to medicine in Edinburgh during Cullen's era. See also Barfoot, M., 'Pedagogy, practice and politics: the Gregory-Bell dispute and the nature of early 19th-century Edinburgh medicine', In Nicolson, M., (ed.) *The changing face of Scotland's health and medicine*, London: Routledge (forthcoming).

29. See Barfoot, M., 'Brunonians under the bed: an alternative to university medicine in Edinburgh in the 1780s'. In Bynum, W.F., Porter, R., (eds), *Brunonianism in Britain and Europe*, London: Wellcome Institute for the History of Medicine, 1988: 22–45.

30. Gregory, J., *Additional memorial to the managers of the Royal Infirmary*, Edinburgh: Murray and Cochrane, 1803: 186–7.

31. Christie, J.R.R., 'Edinburgh medicine in the eighteenth century: the view from the students', *Bull. Soc. Soc. Hist. Med.* 1976; *19*: 13–15.

32. The principal example of this is the contrasting approaches to medicine displayed by Cullen and John Gregory while joint professors of medicine between 1769 and 1773. However the theory and practice chairs were not the only platforms for divergent views. Any professor who had the word 'medicine' in the title of his commission of office could also deliver clinical lectures and, in this capacity, there were ample opportunities to present alternative views on practice. Also, the professor of medicine and anatomy could draw out the special relevance of his subject for the practice of medicine and so challenge views emanating from the practice chair. After John Gregory's death this is precisely what Cullen's chief competitors James Gregory and Alexander Monro *secundus* did.

33. See Bell, W.J., 'Some American students of "that shining oracle of physic" Dr William Cullen of Edinburgh, 1755–1766', *Proc. Am. Phil. Soc.* 1950: *94*: 275–81.

34. The following comment is entirely typical: 'Dr Cullen finished his inimitable course much to the regret of all admirers of great and enlightened views in Medicine. I am rather low upon the occasion, as in all probability I shall never hear that great man again. I wish God, the author of all good, may enable me to apply the instructions I have received from him [and] my other masters for the benefit of my fellow creatures.' See 'Part of the diary of Silas Neville, covering his stay in Edinburgh, 1771–76, also 1781'. EUL Mic M 29 (unpaginated). The passage can also be found in Neville, S., *The diary of Silas Neville 1767–1788*, Ed. Cozens-Hardy, B. London: Oxford University Press, 1950: 216.

35. The debates and dissertations of the Royal Medical Society are well known, but see also Jackson, S.H., *A treatise on medical sympathy, and on the balance and connection of the extreme vessels of the human body*, London: Robson and Clarke, 1787: 120–6. Jackson recounts how he took up an invitation by Cullen at the end of a lecture to submit written objections to any aspect of the doctrine of fever. Cullen replied clarifying his views on febrile sympathy. Jackson remained dissatisfied and stated that his 'turbulent spirit for enquiry into the philosophy of medicine' eventually led him to publish his own views.

36. Risse, G.B., 'Dr William Cullen, Physician, Edinburgh: a consultation practice in the eighteenth century', *Bull. Hist. Med.* 1974: *48*: 338–51.

37. Cullen, W., *A letter to Lord Cathcart, President of the Board of Police in Scotland, concerning the recovery of persons drowned and seemingly dead*, London: Murray, 1774.

38. Cullen's activities as a chemical and agricultural improver fall outside the scope of this paper, but there are some exceptions in the medical sphere as well. See, for example, the draft essays on the preservation of health, hypochondriac disease and the effects of custom, in GUL Cullen MS, box 4, nos. 1–3, 8–13 (new catalogue). Parts of all three are in Cullen's hand and there are also separate transcriptions of the first two in box 6, nos. 11–12. The first was possibly written as a public address; the second was a long consultation letter to his friend and patron, Baron John Maule of Inverkeillor; and the third may have been the source for his institutes lectures on custom, and his son Henry's dissertation, *De Consuetudine*. For a discussion which uses some of this material see Stott, R., 'Health and virtue: or how to keep out of harm's way. Lectures on pathology and therapeutics by William Cullen c. 1770', *Med. Hist.* 1987: *31*: 123–42.

39. Cullen W., 'Lectures on physiology', 2 vols, RCPE MS 16. vol. 2 (unpaginated).

40. Quoted in Thomson, ref. 3. vol. 1: 130.

41. Gregory, J., *Memorial to the managers of the Royal Infirmary*, Edinburgh: Murray and Cochrane, 1800: 209. Gregory went on to applaud this statement as the answer 'of a man of genius, who thoroughly understood his own profession, and the situation in which he was placed'.

42. *Ibid.*, 209–10.

43. Bell, J., *Answer for the junior members of the Royal College of Surgeons of Edinburgh to the memorial of Dr James Gregory*, Edinburgh: Peter Hill, 1800, sect. 1: 52.

44. Gregory, ref. 30: 189.

45. *Ibid.*, 30: 186–93. Gregory used Cullen's *First lines* as his own course textbook. Referring to what he regarded as the more speculative parts of it he commented; 'Those theories I consider as a kind of Apocrypha, allowed to remain between the Canoninical books of the Old and those of the New Testament; which Apocrypha every student is well entitled to believe or to reject, according to the measure of his own understanding and faith. He may be an equally good physician whether he believes it or not.'

46. *Ibid.*, 30: 185–6, where Gregory claimed Cullen's 'Tub', or theory of the nervous system, usually amused the 'Whale' for no less than two-thirds of the 120 lectures, with Cullen 'illustrating very fully, and in a most entertaining manner, many hypothetical theories, about the nature and properties of a supposed nervous fluid or aether; the existence of which still remains to be proved.' Gregory continued: 'He even amused himself and his pupils, by adopting and inculcating some ingenious opinions, never yet established by any competent evidence, concerning the operations of the brain and nerves, and their supposed fluid, in various functions of the body, as for example, in the secretion, preparation, conveyance, and application of nourishment to every part of the body.' Gregory implied that, after friendly hints from colleagues, and the publication of a critical article on 'Aether' in the first edition of the *Encyclopaedia Britannica* (vol. 1: 31–4), Cullen more or less gave up this concept. But see Cullen, ref. 22: 103–8, which indicates he remained committed to the ether-based nervous fluid as an explanatory concept. Also in Cullen, ref. 39, vol. 1 (unpaginated), Cullen explicitly stated that the nutritious fluid of the nerves was not the vehicle of sense and motion.

47. *Ibid.*, 30: 191.

48. Cullen, ref. 14, vol. 1: 363–464. Cullen also inserted parts of them into the expanded preface of the fourth edition of the *First lines*, vol. 1: i–xlviii. An edited version of the section on method, based on Thomson's text, has recently been published. See Cullen, W., 'An introductory lecture to the course on the practice of physic given at Edinburgh University in the years 1768–89', Ed. Passmore, R., *Proc. R. Coll. Phys. Edin.* 1987: *17*: 268–85. It is not known precisely which copies Thomson drew upon. However, the final version in the *Works*, though based on lectures once spoken was probably written out by an amanuensis. Copies of his first actual lecture on the practice of physic course written after 1773 suggest that he not only condensed his opening remarks, he also composed a new introductory lecture for each academic session. See Cullen MSS, GUL Box 3A, nos. 4–6, 12–13, and 16–19.

49. See Christie, J.R.R., 'Ether and the science of chemistry', In Cantor, G.N., M.J.S. Hodge (eds), *Conceptions of ether: studies in the history of ether theories 1740–1900*, Cambridge: Cambridge University Press, 1981: 85–110.

50. Cullen, ref. 14, vol. 1: 398. For a reassessment of this tradition, see Emerson, R.L., 'Conjectural history and Scottish philosophers', In Johnson, D., Ovellette, L. (eds), *Historical Papers 1984/Communications Historiques*, Ottawa: Canadian Historical Association, 1984: 63–90.

51. The best known example is the essay on the history of astronomy by his friend and Glasgow colleague, Adam Smith. See Smith A. *Essays on philosophical subjects*. London: Cadell, 1795: 1–93. Cullen does not use the precise psychological account of the role of the imagination found in this essay. Nevertheless, his account resembles Smith's own in several other respects. In particular, both men laid great stress upon hypotheses and theories as important agents of intellectual change. For a wider discussion see Barfoot M., 'Adam Smith and William Cullen: hypochondriasis and the pathology of the imagination.' In Ross I.S., (ed.) *The legacy of Adam Smith* (forthcoming).

52. Cullen, ref. 14, vol. 1: 366.

53. This was the second revolution of physic from ancient dogmatism to the formal empiricism which Cullen associated with Serapion and others living between 287 BC – 0 AD.

54. Cullen, ref. 14, vol. 1: 374.

55. *Ibid.*, 375.

56. *Ibid.*, 398.

57. *Ibid.*, 401. Cullen chose Sydenham as his exemplary practitioner who, he argued, was the first to show 'there might be a great deal of theory in a man's head without its affecting his practice' (p. 403). Cullen stated that theory in Sydenham's hands was a means of uniting his observations under general headings, and that he was unusual in not looking for facts to confirm his theories. Cullen often presented his own theoretical labours in a similar light.

58. *Ibid.*, 397.

59. *Ibid.*, 414–15.

60. This historical rationale for the organisation of Cullen's physiology lectures has gone largely unnoticed and explains why Cullen devoted so much time to the nervous system at the expense of other subjects.

61. Cullen, ref. 14, vol. 1: 425.

62. A significant group of writers whose methodological positions approach Cullen's in this period are the ether theorists, Robinson, Hartley and Le Sage and the related work of Joseph Priestley. Cullen's own commitment to the nervous ether is a well-known feature of his writings. He probably derived his methodological views about the utility of hypotheses from Robinson and Hartley in the first instance. However, he developed them in a more sophisticated way and did not endorse the

search for facts to prove hypotheses as they advocated. In this respect, his views are closer to Le Sage. For a discussion of these figures in the context of the ether, see Laudan, L., 'The medium and the message: a study of some philosophical controversies about ether', in Cantor, ref. 49: 157–86.

63. Cullen, ref. 14, vol. 1: 438 (transcription). Cullen did not subscribe to the increasingly popular view that Newton never indulged in conjectures. Like his friends Lord Kames, George Martine, and Thomas Melville, he regarded hypotheses subjected to experiment as the Newtonian method. See, for example, Melville, T., 'Observations on light and colours', in [Edinburgh Philosophical Society], *Essays and Observations Physical and Literary*, Edinburgh: Hamilton and Balfour, 1756: 12.

64. Cullen, ref. 17, vol. 1: 7. Cullen's favourite phrase to describe the character of those who published fallacious case histories was 'Grand Observateur, grand Menteur'. See Cullen, W., 'Lectures on medicine', 2 vols, RCPE MS 26, vol. 1, sections 4–5 (unpaginated transcription).

65. For a discussion of Cullen's nosology see Lawrence, ref. 13: 347–72.

66. Cullen, ref. 17, vol. 3: 653–4 (transcription).

67. *Ibid.*, vol. 1: 12–13 (transcription).

68. *Ibid.*, vol. 3: 652 (transcription). This aspect of Cullen's thought was emphasised in an unsigned editorial (Edin. Med. Surg. J. 1832; 38: 384–420), probably by D. Craigie and more fully by him when he completed Thomsons *Life* (ref. 3 vol. 2: 610): 'The spirit of his writings, as his mode of thinking was truly skeptical: that is to say, inquiring rather than doubting; and in the examination and discussion of every subject, one of the first proceedings was to propose the question, How many of the facts stated and believed were worthy of credit, and how many were doubtful and totally unworthy of credit? and on what evidence did each fact, if doubtful, rest?' For two recent discussions of Cullen's method in relation to developments in modern medicine, see Wulff, H.R., 'Scepticism in medicine – 200 years ago and today', *Proc. R. Coll. Phys. Edin.* 1988; *18*: 204–9; Richmond, J., 'Introductory lectures 200 years ago and today', *ibid.*, 209–13.

69. Cullen, ref. 17, vol. 1: 654 (transcription).

70. Cullen, ref 16: 171 (transcription).

71. Cullen, ref 19: 21.

72. For a discussion of the wider significance of necessitarian theories of causal judgement in the Scottish context see Barfoot, M., 'Priestley, Reid's circle and the third organon of human reasoning', in Anderson, R.G.W., Lawrence, C. (eds), *Science, medicine and dissent: Joseph Priestley (1733–1804)*, London: Wellcome/Science Museum, 1987: 81–9.

73. See Cullen, ref. 18, *Institutions*: 7. This point is also made repeatedly in various drafts of Cullen's lectures in his own hand which deal with the nature of causation in medicine. For example, see Cullen, ref. 39, vol. 2 (unpaginated): 'The functions every where run in a Circle of Cause [and] Effect'. Similar views can be found in Melville, ref. 63: 89–90. Cullen also used an example of a man killed by a flying splinter during a naval battle to illustrate how the medical language of 'proximate' and 'remote' causes was used. See Cullen, ref. 64 (RCPE MS 26), vol. 1, section 3 (unpaginated).

74. See Cullen, ref. 39, vol. 2, Lecture 8. Nov 17 1766 (unpaginated): '[W]e know nothing of power and efficiency [and] know it only as a fact that by the contiguity of time [and] place two circumstances or phaenomena are constantly connected together, the first in time and place Cause[,] the other effect.' Cullen did not specifically attribute this view of causation to Hume. In keeping with the majority of his contemporaries, he probably viewed it as a taken-for-granted aspect of explanation in mechanical philosophy. However, it is quite clear that Cullen had read

Hume. In volume one of the same manuscript, he explicitly stated that Hume was the first to distinguish between immediate impressions and recollected ideas.

75. See Cullen, 'Lectures on pathology', 2 vols RCPE MS 28, vol. 2 (unpaginated): 'In many cases the Soul must intervene where our reasoning especially the mechanic must fail.' As this passage suggests, Cullen was prepared to acknowledge a role for the mind or soul and even for spirit in general as ultimate causes. However, he maintained that it was imperative to pursue the chain of causes and effects as far as possible beforehand. As he succintly put it elsewhere: 'Weak heads must get out of the Circle as soon as they ca[n]' (in Cullen, ref. 39, vol. 2).

76. Cullen, ref. 75, vol. 2.

77. For a comparison with Cullen's immediate predecessor and successor to the institutes of medicine chair, see Barfoot, M., 'Knowing the nervous system: conceptions of nervous aetiology in the writings of Whytt, Cullen and James Gregory', in *James Gregory (1753–1821) and Scottish scientific metaphysics 1750–1800*, Edinburgh University: PhD thesis, 1983: 197–263.

78. Cullen, ref. 75, vol. 2 (unpaginated). While Cullen found scepticism with regard to the senses a useful means of exposing false facts and denouncing empiricism as an independent means of acquiring medical knowledge, his own medical discourse was thoroughly realist in tone. Thus he continually utilised a vocabulary of powers, motions and forces when describing properties of the nervous system. He also derived laws of the animal economy expressing the hierarchical relations between those powers, motions and forces.

4

Cullen as clinician: organisation and strategies of an eighteenth century medical practice

GUENTER B. RISSE

To Dr Cullen,
Professor of Physic at Edinburgh

Sir
I suffer since 19 years the greatest torture a poor mortal is able of suffering, and you sir are now the only hope I have left; your great knowledge of physic, and of the human body, for which you are celebrated thro all parts of Europe, flatters me with hopes of your having found out some plant, or mineral in nature that might be of service to me: I have consulted some of the first physicians in Europe, but in vain . . .

Mr Cowmeadow (Berlin Sept, 1 1789)[1]

No portrait of William Cullen can be complete without some reference to his extensive clinical activities, especially during the years in Edinburgh. Thanks to recent work by the Porters, we now have a much better understanding about the ideas and attitudes surrounding the health of eighteenth-century upper and middle class patients.[2] Indeed, we know enough to place Cullen in the context of Georgian medical practice and understand his professional activities conducted in a freewheeling, competitive marketplace. At the other end of the social spectrum, hospital studies such as my work on the Royal Infirmary of Edinburgh have revealed important details of Cullen's approach to poor patients admitted to that charitable institution.[3]

This paper, therefore, will describe and compare two quite different aspects of Cullen's clinical endeavours: his extensive private consultation practice conducted through the mail while living in Edinburgh from about 1755 to 1790,[4] and his management of charity patients admitted to the teaching ward at the Royal Infirmary from 1765 until 1774. The former activities, conducted with a widely scattered clientele of aristocratic and middle class individuals, has been extracted from twenty-one folio volumes of correspondence containing close to three thousand letters preserved at the College of Physicians.[5] All 183 records of cases admitted to the Infirmary teaching ward come from four separate student notebooks, with the bulk of clinical histories copied by Richard

W. Hall, a medical student matriculated at the University of Edinburgh, who walked the Infirmary from 1771 to 1774.[6]

If, in imagination one wandered to another era, in this case the Scottish Enlightenment, one might eventually be deflected from the quaint wonders of contemporary political intrigue, manners and dress, to consider the concrete question of health. Suddenly, one is tempted to return to the present, shuddering at the thought of living at a time when sickness was supposedly much more pervasive than today. Moreover, were medical measures then not almost designed to terrorise the sick with foul-tasting emetics and purges, cruel bloodletting and blisters? For many this remains an alien world of iatrogenic suffering that compounded the misery of illness, creating, as one popular author recently characterised it, the 'age of agony'.[7] Quick to dismiss the past as barbarous, we would conclude our imaginary journey into the past by extolling the virtues of contemporary medicine.

Yet, in spite of ignorance regarding the bodily events of health and disease, medical routines in Cullen's time successfully accomplished the goals which, despite their limitations, all healing systems since the dawn of history have had in common: the ability to recognise and legitimise disability, to make sense of abnormal sensations and appearances through patterns of explanation, to lessen anxiety and uncertainty by providing reassurance, and to supply the means to relieve suffering. For one who had the misfortune to fall ill, this was all that could be expected. An eighteenth-century world teeming with self-styled healers and their conflicting claims created a competitive medical market in which wary but eclectic consumers usually held dominant positions. By this time, the traditional divisions between physician, surgeon and apothecary were breaking down.[8] Cullen, in fact, was actually all three at certain periods of his life. Given the uncertainties of professional competence and contemporary medical knowledge, scepticism and distrust were proper patient responses.

Both for a Scottish aristocrat such as the 3rd Duke of Buccleuch,[9] or for John Turnbull, a lowly Edinburgh weaver,[10] Cullen's medical advice merely supplemented popular domestic initiatives, including dietary changes and self-medication. An affluent patient played an especially active role in the selection of a healer, as well as the management of sickness. Faced with an avalanche of medical advice obtained from personal experience, oral folklore traditions, popular books, pamphlets, and magazines, as well as professional opinions, those feeling ill initiated contact with physicians by calling them to their homes or writing letters demanding written advice. Multiple consultations and opinions were the rule.[11] Through it all, the patient's own history remained the critical piece of information from which diagnostic labels and therapeutic recommendations were carefully negotiated.[12]

In the absence of governmental protection – with the exception of selective royal patronage or regulation by professional bodies such as colleges, then restricted to major urban centres – an eighteenth-century practitioner was forced to rely more on his individual social skills, rather than his medical knowledge, to prosper. Those who, like Cullen, were friendly, discreet and capable of handling demanding and fickle patients, succeeded best. A fledgling physician joined community networks of influence and patronage from which a lucrative private practice could eventually be established.[13] This required high visibility at social events, in clubs and societies, and, in Cullen's case, a willingness to perform charitable service at the Edinburgh Infirmary in connection with his professorial duties at the University.[14]

Private consultation practice

Cullen's epistolary consultation practice increased after he succeeded Robert Whytt in the chair of the institutes of medicine in 1766. However, it was only after John Gregory's death in 1773, when he alone held the chair of the practice of medicine, that Cullen's reputation as the premier clinician of the Edinburgh Medical School was assured.[15] It is not surprising that the volume of letters at this juncture soared almost tenfold and remained high for the remaining two decades of his life, a tribute to his personality and position at the apex of Scotland's, indeed Britain's, medical elite (see figure).[16]

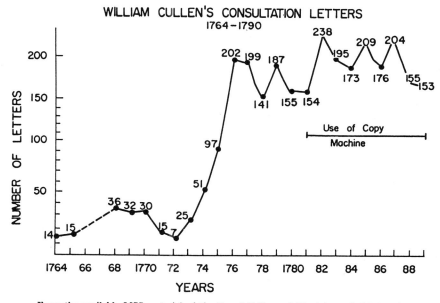

From the available MSS material of the Royal College of Physicians of Edinburgh.

The routines of such a consultation practice reveal that this time-consuming task was handled by Cullen with unparalleled efficiency.[17] Letters addressed to 'Doctor William Cullen, Physician, Edinburgh' were collected by an aide who immediately registered each piece of mail, noting date, source, whether it came from a previous correspondent, patient or practitioner. An early riser, Cullen would read such letters before nine o'clock in the morning and promptly dictate the replies to his secretary-amanuensis before leaving for scheduled patient visits around Edinburgh. 'My hurry has obliged me to employ another hand to transcribe this letter which I hope you'll excuse,' he wrote in 1766.[18] Before completing this daily chore, Cullen would sign the letters and allow his helper to write out on a separate piece of paper the necessary prescriptions accompanying the advice, simply affixing the initials w.c. below the recipes to be entered. The entire reply was then copied for future reference and placed in folios. Most inquiries were indeed answered in this manner within a day.[19]

Then, beginning with a reply dated April 1, 1781, Cullen employed a copying machine invented and patented by James Watt, the famous engineer. It consisted of a page-size press, in which an original ink-written sheet could be placed in contact with thin, chemically prepared copy paper. Both were closely pressed together with the help of a roller. The copy, previously dipped in a solution of vinegar, turned dark brown in those places where it touched the ink, thus rendering an acceptable copy for future reference.[20]

Most letters addressed to Cullen came from Scottish cities and towns, including Aberdeen, Banff, Inverness, Elgin, Paisley, Irvine and Montrose, although a number of correspondents wrote from Carlisle, Berwick-upon-Tweed, Chester, Exeter, Liverpool, Manchester, Newcastle, even Bristol and Southampton, and of course, London. Ireland, the Continent and the New World were represented with requests originating in Dublin, Belfast, Antwerp, Rouen, Genoa, Berlin, Cadiz, New York, New Orleans, and even from the island of Madeira. One patient, writing in 1785 from Boulogne-sur-Mer, told Cullen, 'There is no distance that can prevent us from applying to you when any of us ails'.[21]

Literacy and finances restricted the consultations to upper and middle class patients. Cullen's standard charge for a written opinion was one guinea, but he often left the payment to 'the circumstances and generosity of the patient.'[22] The list of correspondents reads like a Who's Who in Scotland, including the aforementioned Duke of Buccleuch, the Marquess of Tweeddale, the Earl of Dalhousie, the Earl of Hopetoun, the Earl of Selkirk and his Countess, the Earl of Erroll, the Earl of Glasgow, and many others, including clergymen, merchants, and army officers.[23] At times the contact was direct between patient and consultant, but often Cullen also corresponded with physicians attending the sick person, some of them having been his former students. He also dictated private notes directly to the practitioner in charge with specific suggestions and recommendations.[24]

All correspondents naturally viewed Cullen as the final authority. Some personal accounts were quite long – from eight to ten pages – frequently written with the aid of attending practitioners. A twenty-eight page *memoire* written in French and dated October 15, 1785, began with the words 'Comme Le Medecin le plus illustre de l'Europe sa sanction ne peut qu'être desirée avec ordeur'.[25] Another letter from Belfast arrived with what was supposed to be a stool specimen described as 'wonderful fragments with ears or horns, substances like portions of pickled cucumber.' In that particular instance, the patient's maid had spiked the specimen with bird bones to dramatise her mistress's plight.[26] In one 1787 case, Cullen was asked to review five daily pulse readings of a Mrs Murray, all recorded with a stopwatch before and after the patient had spent fifteen minutes exercising on a swing.[27] In several instances Cullen was rewarded with the autopsy reports of cases he had previously treated.

From his correspondence, Cullen emerges as a tactful and compassionate practitioner. In his responses he tried hard to bolster the patients' morale, occasionally even supporting their self-medication if it was not deemed harmful: 'I would willingly think that tho' you are not quite well, you are a good deal better than when I saw you', he wrote to one of them in 1785. 'I can only advise you to persist a little longer in the same remedies and regimen you have hitherto employed'.[29] In his letters, Cullen always stressed that he had carefully considered his patients' accounts, fully understanding their anxieties: 'I am disposed to speak candidly in every case but I cannot possibly be so insensible to the anxiety of the patient and her friend in the present case as not to deliver my opinion very freely and honestly', he wrote to one colleague in 1768.[30] But there were limits. 'I cannot undertake to make her young again', Cullen finally wrote to one consulting practitioner in 1785.[31]

Besides providing reassurance, what could eighteenth-century physicians such as Cullen actually do? From his correspondence ·a contemporary 'art of medicine' emerges that promoted only clinically useful actions acceptable to patients rather than a strict application of prevailing theoretical concerns. At this time it was believed that each confrontation between disease and the individual was a unique experience played out in seemingly endless variations. What mattered above all was the sick person's particular constitution, determined by heredity but always subjected to potentially harmful environmental influences and the effects of lifestyle.[32] Reacting against all injurious outside powers were natural healing forces located within the human organism. Called in to join the struggle, practitioners such as Cullen ostensibly focused on ways to support the patient's endangered constitution and assist the body's natural healing tendencies, while simultaneously warding off or preventing further injuries due to lifestyle and climate.[33] In the contemporary language of a pathophysiology centred on the activities of the nervous system, 'the greater part of a physician's practice consists in exciting, promoting, restraining, and sometimes irritating by art the various operations of nature in the human body,' a most accurate statement made by one of Cullen's colleagues, James Gregory.[34]

From his letters, Cullen emerges both as an overseer of the patient's constitution and a prescriber of the medicinal and physical measures traditionally associated with the relief of symptoms. Diagnosis, in the form of a precise nosological label, was seldom provided. Instead, from a reading of the patients' narratives, Cullen routinely pointed out particular constitutional weaknesses he believed existed in his correspondents. Symptoms were seen as marks of a faulty constitution. The trouble affected the normal functioning of the nervous system. 'I take up his Lordship's care in the view of a nervous system considerably weakened by many shocks which it has received', Cullen revealed to Lord Gardenstone in 1777.[35] For many of his well-to-do male patients, the problem was frequently interpreted as a gouty disposition, a condition with which Cullen, as a sufferer of this disease, was quite familiar. Women, in turn, were quite vulnerable because of the delicacy of their nervous systems which *de facto* subjected them to systemic weakness, the stomach and uterus often bearing the brunt of such perceived and vague constitutional flaws.[36]

But what could really be done? When appropriate, Cullen suggested changes in location and lifestyle for his affluent and indolent clientele. For this purpose, he possessed a detailed knowledge of the local and European climate, insisting that many of his patients spend summers in Scotland and winters in southern England or France.[37] Horseback riding in the countryside and sea voyages provided exercise and fresh air. Cullen was equally familiar with European spas, even providing the temperature and chemical composition of their waters.[38]

The next order of therapeutics comprised dietary prescriptions.[39] Cullen's instructions were usually detailed, with a tendency to reduce the excessive ingestion of meat products and alcoholic beverages in clients notorious for their self-indulgence. This advice usually went beyond Scottish fare. A Prussian official was advised to avoid weak-bodied wines such as Rhenish and most other German wines,[40] while a correspondent in Genoa was informed that chicken and fish dishes in Italy are too rich.

Although he had been a ship's surgeon in his early professional career, Cullen was primarily consulted for medical conditions. Some correspondents sought him out in hopes of receiving advice that would preclude a surgical intervention. Suffering from an urethral stricture, one London patient of John Hunter wrote, 'Mr Hunter in talking of my general complaint is quite the surgeon putting but little faith in the use of inward medicines. He talks of knocking off excrescences in the urethra as a mason would'.[41] Medical treatments, however, often involved venesections, blisters, and setons. Cullen even ordered electrical sparks for patients with muscular weakness or 'obstruction' of the menses.[42]

As for drug treatments, Cullen made sure that the bowels of his sedentary and overnourished patients stayed open with the help of laxatives such as aloe pills and asafetida. However, a stimulating regimen based on the use of several tonics was required for the frequently diagnosed 'constitutional weakness'. This involved the use of Peruvian bark extract, camphor and the powdered leaves of poison hemlock.[43] To improve the gastric tone, impairment of which was believed to be responsible for dyspepsia, Cullen provided soft lozenges or aromatic pills made of cinnamon, ginger and syrup, the so-called saline julep, and aqueous solutions of juniper.[44] For pain, he prescribed opium pills prepared with soap and syrup, or used laudanum, a tincture of the same narcotic, always aware of their habit-forming qualities. In spite of all his efforts, some patients remained dissatisfied with Cullen's advice. 'Agreeable to your directions, I used the nervous infusion for a fortnight which had not the least effect', complained one Mary Forsyte in 1786.[45]

In sum, Cullen's consultation letters deal mostly with wealthy patients considered to possess a fragile constitution that had been compromised by a life of luxury and indolence. These individuals were afflicted most often with chronic complaints for which they sought a second or third opinion through the mail. While responding promptly, Cullen wisely avoided diagnostic distinctions for patients whose conditions he barely knew. Instead, he provided an authoritative agenda for moderate living based on the prevailing ideology of health. His sometimes very precise and detailed advice usually focused more on diet and drink than drugs, and most prescriptions contained mild, well-known botanicals. One can thus argue that the key to Cullen's success was the manner in which he conducted this mail order practice. His patrons were quite important to him, not their diseases. He was attentive, efficient, and always supportive, accompanying his advice with plausible explanations based on a widely accepted constitutional pathology that focused specifically on deficiencies of the nervous system.

Hospital practice in the Royal Infirmary

Shifting attention from famous, wealthy, and educated patients, we must now focus on the plight of Edinburgh's 'deserving poor' who, in the second half of the eighteenth century, were 'desirous of accommo-dation' at the Royal Infirmary of Edinburgh. Like their upper-class counterparts, the poor also played important roles in the expanding medical marketplace and at this time showed a willingness to seek medical advice and even hospital care. In contrast to Cullen's wealthy correspondents, most of the persons requesting admission to the Infirmary suffered from acute conditions, especially fevers. Before being allowed to enter, however, they first had to procure letters of recommendation from hospital subscribers and then present themselves to the Admissions Room, where university professors periodically screened them for possible admittance to the teaching ward.[46]

The existence of this so-called 'clinical' ward went back to 1748 and the efforts of John Rutherford. The unit only remained open during the six months of the academic year, and the professors in charge of it usually divided this duty amongst themselves, each serving three months in rotation. Cullen had begun working at the hospital in 1757 with Whytt and Monro *primus*, then in the 1760s sharing the work with John Gregory. After Gregory's death in 1773, Cullen assumed sole respons-ibility for the teaching ward until 1774.[47] Since attending professors also gave separate clinical lectures, enrolled medical students were allowed to copy the complete medical histories of patients scheduled to be discussed in class. The survival of such student notebooks provides us with the only opportunity to assess contemporary clinical conditions among the sick poor and follow their daily management within the institution.[48]

Hospital cases used in this study came from four different Cullen rotations. A total of 183 Infirmary inmates who were admitted to the teaching ward and managed by Cullen were included. The first patients were seen during the academic years 1763-4 and 1765-6, another contingent in 1772, and finally two groups in 1772-3 and 1773-4.[49] The average age of Cullen's patients was about twenty-five years, women being slightly younger (23.7) than the men (26.5). In this limited sample, females predominated somewhat over males, 55.5 to 44.5 per cent. On average, individuals hospitalised by Cullen remained thirty days in the hospital, including a brief final period for convalescence. Duration of stay was slightly less in women than in men but the difference was insignificant. On discharge, 56 per cent of all patients were labelled 'cured' by Cullen, with females achieving a significantly higher cure rate (over 65 per cent) in comparison with males (44 per cent). The overall mortality rate in Cullen's patients was 6.6 per cent, the rate in men (11 per cent) being significantly higher than that in women (3 per cent).

When these results are compared with those of 800 patients who were admitted to the Infirmary by other medical professors between 1770 and

1800 it is evident that Cullen's case selection and patient management were broadly similar to those obtaining in the Infirmary's teaching ward during the last three decades of the eighteenth century.[50] During his periodic tenure of the teaching ward Cullen seems to have selected a slightly younger population of patients than those chosen over a later period by his colleagues and successors, kept them in the hospital for about a month, but then discharged fewer of them as 'cured'. Cullen also experienced fewer deaths among his patients, perhaps because they were younger and less critically ill.

Patients admitted to the Infirmary's teaching ward constituted the essential 'clinical material' for practical instruction. Indeed Cullen's stated intention was to 'teach the practice of physic by examples'.[51] He was inclined to present diseases of 'a more ordinary appearance' and acute status, believing that they would 'admit of frequent trials in practice' and thus possess greater didactic value.[52] Teaching usually took place during daily rounds, conducted every noon in the teaching ward during his rotation, and supplemented by clinical lectures carried out twice a week, usually on Tuesday and Friday evenings, during the same three months. To attend both events, students needed to purchase admission tickets and, for each clinical lecture, they copied from the master ward journal those cases most likely to be presented in class.[53] Before lecturing, Cullen himself was in the habit of making extensive notes about selected patients whose symptoms, diagnosis, and therapeutic management were to be discussed.[54]

Given the need for accountability in a charitable and public institution such as the Edinburgh Infirmary, diagnostic labels were always required either on admission or at discharge and these were entered in the General Register of Patients.[55] The recorded diagnoses of Cullen's hospital patients ranged widely from fever to dropsy, ague to dyspepsia, and ophthalmia to hysteria. However, the three most commonly identified ailments are fever (61 cases), pectoral complaints (25), and rheumatism (21), comprising nearly 60 per cent of all labels assigned to his patients in the teaching ward. Patients suffering from continuous, as opposed to intermittent, fever were mostly under twenty years of age while those afflicted with respiratory ailments were mainly in their mid- to late twenties with a smaller group in their forties. The classification 'rheumatism' was also given to two separate clusters: teenagers and young adults with acute symptoms and a smaller, older population in their fifties and sixties with chronic complaints. Patients who suffered from fever and respiratory problems stayed hardly three weeks in the hospital, while on the average inmates with rheumatism remained there twice as long.

During his 1772–3 rotation, Cullen accepted twenty-two female patients with fever, suggesting to the students in his lectures that perhaps an epidemic was raging in Edinburgh.[56] A similar situation occurred during the following winter. While the total sample remains small, Cullen's 61 fever patients, 47 female and 14 male, provide a glimpse of his clinical management style with respect to charity cases suffering from acute disease. Given the fact that the cardinal symptoms of fever were difficult to feign in the admission room, (impostors hoping to pass part of the winter in the Infirmary remained a perennial concern of Cullen's),[57] these cases truly record the great clinician in action. The average age of the patients was twenty-two, with the women being slightly younger than the men. At the time of admission, most had been ill for less than a week with half of the men stating that they had received some kind of treatment for their complaints before entering the institution.

Like many of his professional contemporaries, Cullen distinguished two basic types of fevers according to their ostensible clinical character-istics.[58] One kind of febrile illness was called 'inflammatory' fever or *synocha* with general malaise, headaches, flushed face, and a strong pulse. The other was called 'low nervous' fever or *typhus* with a number of gradually evolving nervous symptoms such as drowsiness, muscular tremors, and delirium. In clinical practice however, it was generally difficult to witness such pure nosological entities, and Cullen readily admitted the existence of a 'mixed' form with inflammatory and nervous symptoms which he proceeded to call *synochus*.[59]

Commenting in his 1772–3 clinical lectures, Cullen expressed the opinion that synochus was the most common type of fever then seen in Scotland. He suspected that the condition was acquired through exposure to cold, triggering the action of a weak contagion which alone did not have the power to cause it.[60] 'I have been obliged to form one [opinion] for myself and it is upon my own system that I must proceed', Cullen told his students.[61] Far from being merely a theoretical issue, the distinction between inflammatory and seemingly non-inflammatory fevers was critical for management of the disease. It resulted from Cullen's neuropathological views of the human organism. As with all other ailments, the bodily system was either overexcited and needed to be moderated, or it was weak and required strengthening.[62]

Cullen's synochus fevers, however, were somewhat more complex, since they could alternatively display phases of systemic arousal and depression. If the febrile episode began with complaints of generalised aching, bouts of shivering, a flushed face and full pulse, Cullen would diagnose a truly inflammatory state and order traditional 'anti-phlogistic' measures to calm the body. Conversely, if the presenting symptoms were primarily loss of strength, malaise, anorexia and nausea, and a fast but feeble pulse, all signs of an already weakened system, Cullen would lean towards the diagnosis of a 'nervous' fever requiring a stimulating plan of cure.[63]

According to Cullen, fevers went through three distinct stages of 'fits'. The initial 'cold' phase was dominated by chills and weariness, caused by exhaustion of the nervous system and secondary arterial spasms over the surface of the body. This was followed by a reactive 'hot' stage with manifestations of increased bodily excitability, including higher temperature, pulse, and vascular relaxation. Finally, the third phase of resolution with restoration of normal excitability occurred as patients experienced profuse sweating, lower pulse rate, and return of appetite.[64]

Following admission to his ward, Cullen's first prescription in virtually all fever cases was an emetic. 'I need not point out to you that the use of emetics makes a great part of our practice in fevers', he told his students.[65] In so doing, Cullen followed traditional views about the importance of cleansing all corruptible matter from an alimentary canal perceived to be weakened by disease. This was especially true in fevers, with nature expressing the disorder through symptoms of anorexia, nausea, and at times, vomiting.[66] By using emetics, Cullen also hoped by art to sufficiently affect the body's inherent excitability so that the fever would quickly shift from the cold to the hot fit phase and thus accelerate the natural healing process.[67] Cullen's rationale for the employment of emetics therefore was based on a combination of traditional humoral and newer neuropathological views. The popularity of this approach can be seen from the clinical histories under scrutiny. Indeed 85 per cent of Cullen's patients in our infirmary sample, 91 per cent of the women and 64 per cent of the men, received repeated doses of such a drug, usually tartar emetic.[68]

Once the manifestations of fever were fully established, Cullen merely let the patients rest, provided liquids or a 'low diet' and if needed, kept their bowels open with the help of purgatives or enemas. Hospital physicians were indeed cautious about giving food, especially when the patients claimed to have no appetite because of their illness and the effects of nauseating drugs. Moreover, if the stomach did not function well, practitioners were fearful of turning ordinary fevers into 'putrid' types through the prescription of heavier food containing meat. To preclude such an eventuality, Cullen and others prescribed great quantities of diluted, acid fruit drinks considered to possess antiseptic qualities required to prevent the gastric putrefaction.[69]

Pointing out the diurnal fluctuations of pulse and temperature, Cullen firmly believed that fevers went through some regular sequences. More important, he strongly supported the Hippocratic notion of 'critical days'.[70] Although he had problems fixing the onset of a fever – the patient's history was frequently held to be unreliable – Cullen argued that the first crisis occurred on the fourth day of the illness with gradual remission until a new crisis developed on the seventh, usually about the time patients sought admission to the hospital. In most instances, the next critical developments were expected to occur on the fourteenth and seventeenth days; remission usually followed thereafter as the patient's body temperature, sleep, and appetite returned to normal, signalling convalescence and total recovery before the twenty-first day.[71]

Convinced that profuse sweating was a natural way for the body to expel unwanted matter, Cullen between crises often tried to help nature by giving some medications to promote sweat. Perspiration was viewed as a stimulating procedure, frequently enhanced by the application of heat in the form of baths and fomentations, or by wearing flannel shirts.[72] In an institutional setting short of nurses, considerable pressure was therefore put on the auxiliary personnel available to help with the baths. In the patient sample, more than a third of the Infirmary patients received diaphoretic drugs, women almost three times as often as the men.

Another stimulating method of treatment popular with Cullen was the production of blisters, deliberately created at selective body locations through the application of irritating substances conveyed in adhesive dressings or plasters.[73] While Cullen remained sceptical concerning their stimulating qualities, he firmly maintained that blisters would exert a systemic, antispasmodic effect, easing the transition from the cold to the hot stage of the fever.[74] In the fever group, more than a third of the patients were blistered, with women nearly twice as often as the men. Because of pain and the danger of secondary infection, most patients dreaded the application of such blisters, often refusing them outright and leaving the hospital to avoid them. Women were especially concerned if the blisters were created on their breasts.

Postulating that 'the use of opium was commonly hurtful', Cullen refrained from providing it too often.[75] He therefore substituted analgesic draughts containing other narcotics such as aconite, belladonna, and hemlock. In the sample under study, one third of the female patients received them, but only one male, perhaps because it was widely assumed that women's constitutions and the delicacy of their nervous systems made them more sensitive to pain. Almost absent from Cullen's regimen was the use of alcoholic beverages, especially wine, which he omitted entirely from the women's diet although other Edinburgh professors frequently prescribed it. At that time, the employment of alcohol was justified for its presumed stimulating effects and many Infirmary practitioners prescribed claret, a light, red wine imported from France, served primarily during the convalescent period diluted with water or milk.[76]

If the presenting symptoms suggested inflammation, Cullen would resort to bleeding, primarily venesection. Age considerations and the patient's complexion entered into that decision.[77] If patients displayed symptoms of weakness such as fainting spells or dizziness, the bleeding was proscribed. In the sample, 52 per cent of Cullen's patients were bled, women again in higher proportion (62) than men (32). The usual amount extracted was said to be eight ounces (about 225 ml) sometimes repeated once or twice in subsequent days by checking the fullness of the pulse as well as the crust formed over the removed blood sitting in the bleeding bowl. Under Cullen's management, venesections averaged a total of twelve ounces per patient until the perceived inflammation subsided. The exception was one seventeen year old female patient who also had a cough and swollen ankles. After already having been bled thirty-five ounces (about 1.1 litre) by Cullen over a period of seven days, a note in her chart indicated that during a prescribed eight-ounce venesection 'blood stopped from flowing when four ounces were drawn'. In spite of this more drastic treatment, the patient recovered fully and was transferred to another hospital ward for her convalescence after Cullen's rotation had ended.[78]

In the end, all of Cullen's fever cases seemed to recover, most of them officially discharged from the Infirmary as 'cured' after an average stay of only twenty-four days, (for the women twenty-two days, the men twenty-seven days, almost a week longer). In the clinical histories, many patients were said to be 'convalescing' during their last days in the institution. For the first time, they now received a full diet containing some meat in the form of beef tea, boiled or roasted beef, mutton, or chicken, both for dinner and supper. In the final analysis, Cullen had, as he often declared, 'acquitted himself tolerably well', although, as he admitted to his students, 'I am not ashamed to say that I do fail in judgment and I shall never hide a doubt with regard to a doctrine I advance or a practice I follow.[79]

Comparison of Cullen's private and hospital practices

Sharp contrasts can be observed between Cullen's mail-order practice and patient management at the Edinburgh Infirmary. Perhaps comparisons are unfair, since in the former instance he was primarily dealing with chronic ailments while in the hospital, patients were acutely ill. Moreover, the bulk of Cullen's correspondents lived outside Edinburgh and their sickness had to be interpreted from written accounts, not always a dependable type of information. This mode of practice suggested an extra dose of caution and less aggressive prescribing of drugs. The hospital practice, on the other hand, involved direct contact with the patients and therefore a more decisive hands-on approach.

A few observations and conclusions are, nevertheless, in order. In his handling of correspondence, Cullen, the foremost medical nosologist of his time,[80] frequently eschewed precise diagnostic labels. While in his textbooks and lectures he repeatedly proclaimed symptoms as being signposts of specific diseases, in his letters Cullen categorised them as merely 'marks of a faulty constitution'. From the correspondence, one can observe a narrower prognostic and therapeutic approach tailored to the individual patient. The intent is clear; Cullen's patrons were important, not their diseases.[81] Thus, Cullen assumed the role of protector of body and mind, monitoring and adjusting the lifestyles of the rich and famous.

In the Edinburgh Infirmary, Cullen's approach had to be different. Bureaucratic constraints and didactic needs forced early diagnostic labelling. This was followed by a much more aggressive management routine that paid less attention to the individual constitutions of the lower-class patient. After all, these individuals were believed to be more robust. Hence, in this institutional setting, the patient was less important than the disease. Even admission to the teaching ward was predicated on Cullen's assessment of a case as an appropriate example of a disease to be studied during his teaching rotation. Subsequent medical interventions tended to follow textbook recommendations with only minor adjustments based on the individual evolution of a given disease, variations which Cullen explained to his students in the clinical lectures.

If we apply the litmus test of venesection to Cullen's disparate patient populations, the contrasts in therapy are significant. In his consultation letters, Cullen was conservative about bleeding, only occasionally recommending the withdrawal of four to six ounces, perhaps to be repeated in one or two days. 'Venesection is powerful but I would not wish to practice it often', Cullen wrote to one of his correspondents, indicating that 'I am certain it contributes to induce a plethoric state'. Paradoxically, instead of the usual fears of weakening delicate wealthy patients through bleeding, Cullen's statement implies that he expected his well-nourished clients to make up more than the medically ordained losses. In the Infirmary, however, Cullen did not seem to harbour the same reservations. More than half of his fever cases had to submit to venesections, the total amount of blood withdrawn from each patient averaging thirteen ounces. In comparison with his male patients, Cullen's female patients endured a significantly higher percentage of all forms of treatment, including venesection.

What can we conclude from the surviving documentation? In his letters and lectures, Cullen undoubtedly emerges as a friendly, disciplined, but cautious practitioner. At the Edinburgh Infirmary, he was therapeutically more aggressive, viewing inherently more hardy charity patients as useful clinical material for his professional advancement and teaching. He also relished exposing malingerers and in general distrusted patients' and nurses' reports. Yet, compared to the treatment employed by some of his contemporaries, the therapeutic measures used by Cullen carried a lesser risk of producing adverse effects. As he told the students, 'I have a rule in practice that I seldom push a remedy that may do harm . . . I would rather let a disease kill a patient than kill him by my medicine'.[82]

At times, on a visit to paying customers, Cullen would also inquire about the fate of his former Infirmary patients. Somewhat less than the 'oracle of physic' his students made him out to be, Cullen to his credit would make no bones about his own shortcomings. 'Some of my colleagues tell me that I am imprudent in telling you my faults', he disarmingly admitted.[83] On balance, Cullen's tact and experience carried him to the top of the eighteenth-century medical pyramid. Unquestionably, this enthusiastic teacher and sceptical practitioner exemplified the best of contemporary clinical medicine in Edinburgh.

Notes and references

1. 'Letters to Dr Cullen', 1755–90, 17 vols. Royal College of Physicians of Edinburgh, Cullen MS 31, vol. 16, letter to Cullen dated 1 September 1789 (filing is in chronological order). Although most of the letters in this MS collection are from correspondents seeking Cullen's medical opinion, some are copies of Cullen's letters of reply. This collection also contains a small number of letters and papers which are unrelated to Cullen's consultation practice.

2. D. and R. Porter, *Patient's Progress; Doctors and Doctoring in Eighteenth-Century England*, Stanford, CA: Stanford University Press, 1989.

3. G.B. Risse, *Hospital Life in Enlightenment Scotland; Care and Teaching at the Royal Infirmary of Edinburgh*, Cambridge and New York: Cambridge University Press, 1986.

4. A partial analysis of this practice can be found in G.B. Risse, 'Doctor William Cullen, Physician, Edinburgh: a consultation practice in the eighteenth century', *Bull. Hist. Med.* 48(1974): 338–51.

5. 'Consultation letters from Dr Cullen', 1768–89, 21 vols. R.C.P.E. Cullen MS 30. These leather-bound folio volumes contain copies of most of the letters which Cullen wrote in reply to requests for medical advice. The letters are filed in chronological order.

6. 'Clinical Cases and Reports by Drs Monro *primus*, Cullen and Whyte', 1763–5, MSS Collection, Royal College of Physicians, London; and 'William Cullen, Clinical Cases and Reports taken at the Royal Infirmary of Edinburgh', in R.W. Hall, 'Dr. Cullen', vols. 1–3, 1771–4, MSS Collection, National Library of Medicine, Bethesda.

7. G.R. Williams, *The Age of Agony: the Art of Healing c. 1700–1800*, London; Constable, 1975.

8. For a useful analysis of the contemporary medical profession in Britain, see I. Loudon, *Medical Care and the General Practitioner, 1750–1850*, Oxford: Clarendon Press, 1986, especially pt 1.

9. The 3rd Duke of Buccleuch (1746–1812) was governor of the Royal Bank of Scotland and first president of the Royal Society of Edinburgh from 1783 until his death.

10. John Turnbull, aged 32, was admitted to the teaching ward of the Edinburgh Infirmary on 2 December 1773 with a rheumatic complaint. Cullen remained in charge of his treatment until the patient was discharged five weeks later on 5 January 1774, ostensibly 'cured'. See Cullen, n.6 above 1773–4 vol.3.

11. Porter and Porter, n. 2 above, pt II, pp. 33–69. For more detail concerning patients' experience of illness based on their own writings,

see D. and R. Porter, *In Sickness and in Health, the British Experience 1650–1850*, London: Fourth Estate, 1988.

12. S.J. Reiser, 'Examination of the Patient in the Seventeenth and Eighteenth Centuries', in *Medicine and the Reign of Technology*, Cambridge and New York: Cambridge University Press, 1978, pp. 1–22.

13. Porter, n.2 above, pt III, pp. 117–44.

14. Beginning in 1757, Cullen gave clinical lectures to medical students attending the Edinburgh Infirmary. He shared this responsibility with Drs Robert Whytt and Alexander Monro *primus*. This meant that all three professors also shared the supervision of the teaching ward with its day-to-day management of between twelve and twenty patients.

15. For a biographical sketch see R.W. Johnstone, 'William Cullen', *Med. Hist.* 3 (1959): 33–46, and the entry 'William Cullen' in Robert Chambers' *A Biographical Dictionary of Eminent Scotsmen*, Glasgow 1855, vol. 2, pp. 18–37. Cullen's biographer, John Thomson, received the physician's papers from the family following the death of Lord Robert Cullen, a son of William, who had originally intended to carry out the assignment himself. Thomson went on to write a 2-vol. work entitled *An Account of the Life, Lectures, and Writings of William Cullen, M.D.*, Edinburgh: W. Blackwood & Sons, 1859.

16. All surviving replies by Cullen filed in the 21 folio vols (see n.5 above) were individually counted. All but three of the vols have a patient index, prepared to help Cullen and his assistant in those instances when he needed to review the previous correspondence.

17. For a brief description of this correspondence see J.D. Comrie, 'An Eighteenth-Century Consultant', *Edinburgh Med. J.* 32 (1925): 17–30. Comrie reproduces seven letters concerned with smallpox inoculation, hysteria, dyspepsia and other conditions. One letter came from James Boswell, another from John Hunter.

18. Letter from Cullen dated 10 May 1766 (n.1 above, vol. 1).

19. Details of Cullen's routine can be found in an anonymous letter in the Thomson/Cullen MSS Collection, Glasgow University Library. The document was probably obtained by Dr Thomson who, in preparation for his biographical work, strenuously solicited testimonials and recollections of Cullen's activities. Cullen mentioned his prescription writing habits in a letter dated 4 July 1789. Corrections in his own handwriting can be noted on numerous occasions, especially if such a letter went to an important consultant or prominent patient.

20. Watt's invention is mentioned in H.W. Dickinson, *James Watt, Craftsman and Engineer*, Cambridge: University Press, 1935, pp. 115–18. During the latter part of 1779 Watt described his copying machine in some detail to Cullen's friend and successor to the chair of chemistry in Edinburgh, Joseph Black. As a result of an intense publicity campaign among bankers and members of Parliament, Watt was able to sell more than 150 of his devices in the first year. Black, writing to Watt from Edinburgh on 7 January 1780 about the copying machine, mentions Cullen as a potential customer 'to whom it will be extremely useful'. (See E. Robinson and D. McKie, eds, *Partners in Science, Letters of James Watt and Joseph Black*, London: Adams and Dart, 1970, p. 75.

21. Letter to Cullen, dated 5 August 1785 (n.1 above, vol. 12).

22. Letter from Cullen dated 16 September 1789 (n.5 above, vol. 21).

23. For details concerning Cullen's aristocratic patients see G.E. Cockayne, *The Complete Peerage of England, Scotland, Ireland, Great Britain and the United Kingdom*, new revised and enlarged edition, 13 vols., ed. V. Gibbs, London, 1910.

24. A private note in a letter from Cullen dated 23 September 1779 (n.5 above, vol. 12) informed the attending physician of Cullen's suspicion

that the patient was indeed suffering from phthisis and should be carefully monitored.

25. Letter to Cullen dated 15 October 1785 (n.1 above, vol. 12).
26. Letter to Cullen dated 3 November 1783 (*ibid.*, vol. 10).
27. Letter to Cullen dated 20 March 1787 (*ibid.*, vol. 14). The patient had previously complained of chest pains. The observations on her pulse rate were recorded by her husband in an enclosed letter dated 27 February 1787.
28. Letter to Cullen dated 8 May 1782 (*ibid.*, vol. 9).
29. Letter from Cullen dated 1 August 1785 (n.5 above, vol. 18).
30. Letter to Cullen dated 25 May 1768 (n.1 above, vol. 1).
31. Letter from Cullen dated 3 September 1785 (n.5 above, vol. 18).
32. 'Your nervous system, originally weak, has received some shocks and your complaint is entirely from disordered nerves affecting both mind and body', from a letter written by Cullen to a patient on 7 December 1778 (*ibid.*, vol. 11).
33. 'You have got into a very relaxed state of nerves . . . I suspect your constitution originally has been strong but intemperance has been especially to blame and your first step is to avoid this for the future.' Letter from Cullen dated 10 February 1777 (*ibid.*, vol. 8).
34. James Gregory, *Additional Memorial to the Managers of the Royal Infirmary*, Edinburgh, 1803, pp. 412–13.
35. Letter from Cullen dated 30 August 1777 (n.5 above, vol. 9).
36. In one undated letter Cullen ascribed the patient's hysteria to 'nervous atrophy', and 'depending upon a peculiar irritability in her own and her family's constitution. That this should produce some irregularity in the uterine discharges is what might be expected'. (*ibid.*, vol. 13).
37. Letter from Cullen dated 7 September 1785 (*ibid.*, vol. 18). In another letter, dated 13 April 1779, Cullen declared that 'the air on the coast of Fife is as pure as can be, but when the wind sets in from the northeast as it does in April–May, the air is very bleak' (*ibid.*, vol. 11).
38. Letter from Cullen dated 15 October 1784 (n.1 above, vol. 11).
39. See William Cullen, 'Therapeutics', in 'Institutes of Medicine, lecture notes,' Edinburgh 1772 (MSS Collection, National Library of Medicine, Bethesda, vol. 7, p. 7).
40. Letter from Cullen to William Baylies in Berlin concerning the health of Mr Heynitz, dated 15 October 1784 (n.1 above, vol. 11).
41. Letter to Cullen dated 6 June 1782 (*ibid.*, vol. 9).
42. In a letter dated 21 September 1777 (*ibid.*, vol. 4) one patient spoke of his own 'electrifying machine'. In a letter dated 22 January 1779 (n.5 above, vol. 11) to a Miss A.B. suffering from menstrual irregularities, Cullen suggested the application of numerous daily electrical shocks through the loins.
43. A representative regimen is that for Lord Gardenstone in a letter dated 30 August 1777 (n.5 above, vol. 9).
44. Letter from Cullen dated 7 August 1776 (ibid., vol. 8).
45. Letter to Cullen dated 19 May 1786 (n.1 above, vol. 13).
46. See Risse, n.3 above, pp. 60–118.
47. *Ibid.*, pp. 242–9. Cullen's departure is documented in the minutes of the meeting held by the managers of the Royal Infirmary dated 17 November 1774. I am indebted to Dr Barfoot for this information.
48. *Ibid.*, appendix A, pp. 296–301.
49. See n.6 above.
50. Risse, n.3 above, pp. 90–2 and chapters 4 & 5 *passim*.
51. William Cullen, *Clinical Lectures Delivered in the Years 1765 and 1766*, London: Lee & Hurst, 1797, p. 1.
52. William Cullen, 'Clinical Lectures,' 1772–3, 4 vols. Royal College of Physicians of Edinburgh, Cullen MS 4, vol. 1, p. 29.

53. Risse, n.3 above, pp. 242–55.
54. Thomson, n.15 above, vol. 1, pp. 107–8.
55. Risse, n.3 above, pp. 43–56.
56. Case of Hannah Cameron, age 46, admitted to the Infirmary on 5 March 1772; in Cullen, n.6 above, *1771–2*, vol. 1.
57. See for example the case of Thomas Williamson in Cullen, n.52 above vol. 1, p. 60.
58. In the 1730s John Huxham had already distinguished two basic categories of continuous fevers: the 'inflammatory', and 'low nervous'. Such a differentiation had important therapeutic implications. See John Huxham, *An Essay on Fevers and their Various Kinds*, London: Austen, 1750. For further details see G.B. Risse, 'Typhus fever in eighteenth-century hospitals: new approaches to medical treatment', *Bull. Hist. Med.* 59 (1985): 176–95.
59. 'There are only three kinds of continuous fevers. The inflammatory or what we call *synocha*. The nervous fever or what we call *typhus* and a species that is always a combination of these two to which we have confined the appellation of *synochus*. It is this last one which is most frequent in the country and particularly at the present season', Cullen, n.52 above, *1772–3*, vol. 1, pp. 129–30. Cullen's nosological categories were originally published in his *Synopsis Nosologiae Methodicae*, Edinburgh, 1769.
60. 'Contagions are not powerful without concurring causes; here our contagions are very rarely powerful enough to do it without the concurrent application of cold, and it is evident that such is the fever we speak of', Cullen, n.52 above, vol. 1, p. 131.
61. *Ibid.*, p. 132.
62. For a more detailed discussion see Risse, n.3 above, pp. 177–83.
63. Cullen, n.52 above, vol. 1, p. 136.
64. See William Cullen, 'Of Fevers', in *First Lines of the Practice of Physic*, new ed., Edinburgh: C. Eliot, 1786, vol. 1, pp. 65–85. For a useful overview of contemporary ideas about fever see the article 'Febris' in Bartholomew Parr, *The London Medical Dictionary*, Philadelphia: Mitchell, Ames & White, 1819, vol. 1, pp. 642–54.
65. Cullen, n. 52 above, vol. 1, p. 136.
66. *Ibid.*, vol. 1, pp. 136–7.
67. As Cullen told his students, 'the whole affair of the exhibition of emetics may be explained upon another footing than merely by the throwing out of the morbid matter', then going into a lengthy discussion about how the atony of the stomach was linked by sympathy to the skin vessels (*ibid.*, vol. 1, pp. 138–40).
68. Cullen frequently declared that he liked to 'wash out the stomach' with tartar emetic, although one had to monitor the drug's 'tendency to run off by stool'. Fulfilling the dual goals of vomiting and purging, tartar emetic was an attractive remedy, but its effects were often unpredictable and physicians tended needlessly to increase the dosage (*ibid.*, vol. 1, pp. 181 and 189).
69. See Thomson, n.15 above, vol. 1, pp. 606–8.
70. 'I am of the opinion that there is a constant tendency in nature for fevers to observe regular movements, and I have been more frequently able to observe them distinctly than that I have missed them' (Cullen, n.52 above, vol. 1, p. 199).
71. Cullen's extensive discussion about 'critical days' using his Infirmary patients as examples is contained in the lecture notes (*ibid.*, vol. 1, pp. 198–216; vol. 2, pp. 217–20).
72. For a summary see Risse, n.3 above, pp. 196 and 212–13. Details can be found in Andrew Duncan, *Elements of Therapeutics*, 2nd ed., Edinburgh: Drummond, 1773, vol. 2, pp. 23–33. According to Cullen,

total immersion in hot water could not 'be administered with any convenience and propriety in hospitals if the patients were not ambulatory' (Cullen, n.52 above, vol. 1, p. 164).

73. See 'Blisters' in Parr, n.64 above, vol. 1, pp. 254–6.
74. Cullen, n.52 above, vol. 1, p. 150.
75. *Ibid.*, vol. 1, pp. 153–4.
76. The omission of wine prescriptions is not too surprising, given Cullen's belief that alcohol was more of a sedative than a stimulant (See pp. 181–83 of this book).
77. In one case, Cullen told the students that 'flushing of the face directed me to guard against the determination of the blood to her head, so that I ordered her to be blooded for three days successively' (Cullen, n.52 above, vol. 1, p. 187).
78. Case of Christian Crais, admitted 4 December 1773, in Cullen, n.6 above, vol. 3. This patient remained in the hospital for more than two months.
79. Cullen, n.52 above, vol. 4, p. 209.
80. Lester S. King, 'Nosology', in *The Medical World of the Eighteenth Century*, Chicago: University of Chicago Press, 1958, pp. 193–226. See also R.E. Kendell, 'William Cullen's *Synopsis nosologiae methodicae*', in this book, pp. 216–233.
81. See N.D. Jewson, 'Medical Knowledge and the Patronage System in 18th Century England', *Sociology* 8 (1974): 369–85.
82. Cullen, n.52 above, vol. 3, p. 541.
83. *Ibid.*, vol. 4, p. 339.

5

Cullen and the nervous system

W . F . B Y N U M

The importance of the nervous system in William Cullen's medical writings and teaching is well known, nor was this simply a phenomenon of his Edinburgh period. Robert Wallace, the Glasgow surgeon, recalled to Cullen's biographer, John Thomson, that Cullen sometimes gave to his Glasgow students 'a manuscript half-sheet, to be copied and circulated from one to another; and in his lectures has delivered the same opinions with regard to the Theory of Fever, the Humoral Pathology, and the Nervous System, which have since appeared in his writings'.[1] Cullen himself has also alerted us to the centrality of the nervous system when, in a much-quoted comment, he insisted that 'In a certain view, almost the whole of the diseases of the human body might be called NERVOUS'.[2] Even this sentiment was not created by Cullen: his colleague Robert Whytt said much the same thing some years before ('There are few disorders which may not in a large sense be called nervous');[3] in the late seventeenth century Thomas Sydenham had pronounced hysteria and similar disorders as constituting half the chronic diseases affecting human beings. Early in the nineteenth century, Thomas Trotter, who studied in Edinburgh towards the end of Cullen's reign there, raised the ante to two-thirds in describing the percentage of nervous disorders with which he believed civilised society was afflicted.[4]

'All', 'almost the whole', 'two-thirds' 'half': even the mildest 'half' sounds a bit hyperbolic. Nevertheless, that Sydenham, Whytt, Cullen and Trotter – four sober and respected clinicians over a period of just over a century – could make such judgements suggests, at the least, that the long eighteenth century took the nervous system seriously as a cause of disease and, by implication, as an essential constituent of health. That hysteria was for Sydenham not quite the *nervous* disorder that it became for the doctors of Whytt's and Cullen's generation, is beside the point, or the perception. There were earlier authorities for those who in the middle third of the eighteenth century reconceptualised the physiological nature of disease, a process to which Cullen contributed but hardly initiated. Even Cullen's first major – and in many ways best – analyst, never claimed for him the dubious title of midwife of the nerves. John Thomson's judgement was that:

> In this country, it was Dr. Cullen who first perceived the value of the doctrine of the Nervous Pathology introduced by [Friedrich] Hoffmann; and from the time he began to lecture on medicine in Glasgow, he not only adopted that doctrine, but uniformly endeavoured to render to the memory and writings of its author that commendation and applause to which the importance of his improvements in pathology, and in the descriptions of diseases, and his candour and impartiality to others, gave him so just a claim.[5]

Whether 'this country' meant for Thomson 'Scotland' or Great Britain, is unclear; but even in Scotland itself, Cullen's preoccupation with the nervous system was shared by most of the other leading medical teachers of his generation, including Alexander Monro *secundus*, Robert Whytt and John Gregory. Whytt's work in particular is impressive not just for its depth and subtlety, but for the way in which he integrated experimental work and clinical observations. Unlike Cullen, Whytt occupies a prominent place in the scholarly assessment of the history of neurophysiology. For instance, in Neuburger's *Historical Development of Experimental Brain and Spinal Cord Physiology before Flourens*, Cullen rates one brief mention in a footnote, along with other medical teachers who perpetuated error; Whytt is expounded as Haller's major rival in the mid-eighteenth century.[6] Cullen gets no reference at all in Clarke and O'Malley's *Human Brain and Spinal Cord*, whereas Whytt receives several passing references and two extended discussions.[7] In Clarke and Jacyna's more recent *Nineteenth-Century Origins of Neuroscientific Concepts*, Whytt is a major background figure, Cullen one of only passing interest.[8] Even John Spillane's more neurologically orientated *Doctrine of the Nerves* devotes twelve pages to Whytt; Cullen gets just over two, almost half of which is taken up with plates.[9] 1991 is the 225th anniversary of Whytt's death: maybe a commemorative symposium would be in order.

Thomson dates Cullen's fascination with the 'Nervous Pathology' to his Glasgow days, although his publications on the topic all come from his Edinburgh period. I know of no work which seeks to trace the origin and development of Cullen's ideas about the nervous system; indeed Cullen is usually presented historically as a static thinker. We need not agree with the verdict of Garrison that 'Sir William Hamilton was perilously near the truth when he said that Cullen did not add a single new fact to medical science' to accept that the nature of Cullen's writings makes it difficult to trace anything as precise as unit ideas.[10] In addition, it can be argued that, at least until very recently, our historical Cullen was largely derived from John Thomson. This is no bad thing; his

Life of Cullen strikes me as one of the best books ever written on eighteenth-century medicine. It is also a very scarce book whose facsimile reproduction would be welcome. Thomson's companion edition of Cullen's *Works* is equally valuable, but it was a distillation of Cullen's writings – published and manuscript – from various periods, put together in a coherent and intelligent way, but perhaps encouraging lazy historians like myself to rely too much on it.

If even Thomson relegates Cullen to the relatively modest role of imparting a system of neuropathology which originated on the Continent, and more recent commentators find it difficult to specify much in the way of particular features to Cullen's writings on the nervous system, what are we left with? These are two things of particular relevance, I think. First, Cullen's reflection of and partici- pation in a much broader cultural phenomenon whereby notions of class, gender, and order – both natural and social – were expressed by reference to the nervous system. Second, an interesting and largely consistent integration of his exposition of the functions of the nervous system within the *Institutes of Medicine* with the much more nosological and therapeutic concerns of his *First Lines of the Practice of Physic*. What Cullen taught, I shall suggest, was not so much the physiology and pathology of the nervous system, but a rather different vision of a single and ultimately indivisible neuro-muscular system.

I shall concentrate on the latter theme, but must first remind you of the growing body of historical literature concerned with what Lawrence has called 'the nervous system and society'.[11] In its simplest terms, this describes the shift from the vascular pathology of Boerhaave to the neuropathology of the mid-century. A good deal of this literature has focused on the Scottish Enlightenment, and on Cullen and his colleagues not as isolated medical men but as active participants in the more general intellectual concerns of the age. Lawrence's Ph.D. thesis was entitled *Medicine as Culture*.[12] Despite Cullen's rather defensive tone when he deals with what could be called metaphysical issues ('When I have considered [the writings of Aristotle, Descartes and Leibniz] as well as I can, I cannot perceive that they have the least effect or influence in explaining any thing'[13]) he was an intimate of David Hume and Adam Smith, and his own philosophical and theological views were clearly influenced by this friendship.[14]

Neurophysiological notions such as sensibility and sympathy also enjoyed much broader cultural ramifications and connotations, and the cult of the 'man of feeling' not only provided novelists, playwrights and poets with material, it also provided doctors with patients.[15] Women were especially susceptible to this cluster of nervous disorders, since their nervous systems were delicate and highly strung. 'One hour's intense thinking wastes the spirits more in a Woman, than six in a Man', opined one of Bernard de Mandeville's characters.[16] Country bumpkins, labourers and, in general, the vulgar, rarely thought and so were relatively immune from loss of spirit. Nervous disorders were the price to be paid for the refinements of civilisation, but also, James Makittrick Adair insisted in 1786, the result of fashion:

> Upwards of thirty years ago, a treatise on nervous diseases was published by my quondam learned and ingenious preceptor, Dr. Whytt, professor of physick, at Edinburgh. Before the publication of this book, people of fashion had not the least idea that they had nerves; but a fashionable apothecary of my acquaintance, having cast his eye over the book, and having been often puzzled by the enquiries of his patients concerning the nature and causes of their complaints, derived from thence a hint, by which he readily cut the Gordian knot – '*Madam, you are nervous*'; the solution was quite satisfactory, the term became fashionable, and spleen, vapours, and hyp, were forgotten.[17]

Adair's account possesses in charm what it lacks in historical subtlety, and nor is the dating to the 1780s of an 'upsurge of interest in nerves' by Hunter and Macalpine very satisfactory, even if, as they suggest, the publication in 1783 of the (enlarged) third edition of Cullen's *First Lines*, contained a full discussion of the class of diseases he had first called the neuroses.[18]

The coining of this term by Cullen is probably his single most commonly remembered deed, though I doubt if he would have held it in such high esteem, especially since he was a neologistic conservative, insisting on his aversion to the introduction of new names for diseases.[19] Nor, unsurprisingly, were Cullen's neuroses ours. The concept has undergone a complicated process of evolution over the past two centuries; ironically, its meaning was probably just as precise and consistent for Cullen as it is in our age of anxiety.

By the time of the publication of the third edition of the *First Lines*, the earlier age of 'nerves' was in full swing, and I would not want to deny to Cullen a role in it. The ascription of physical and physiological differences (between men and women, between Europeans and savages, between the members of the Edinburgh clubs and those who served them) and the social and moral implications (about the 'naturalness' of the hierarchies between gender, class, race, or nation) were so widespread that, it could be argued, Cullen must have subscribed to them. I am sure he did, but it is exceptionally difficult to construct anything that we might call a sociology or an anthropology from Cullen's published writings. Perhaps his interest in nosology led him to minimize the individual and idiosyncratic. Alternatively, it could be suggested that he was a reluctant and contingent nosologist and that Cullen, the Humean sceptic, doubted the naturalness of disease categories. Certainly he was not given to easy generalizations, and his favourite explanatory categories seems to have been the environmental ones of heat and cold, and the individual one of habit or custom.[20] For Cullen, cautious qualification was the order of the day.

Consider, for instance, his comment, already quoted, that 'almost the whole of the diseases of the human body might be called NERVOUS'. This is immediately followed by the sensible caveat: 'But there would be no use for such a general appelation', a caveat John Brown would have done well to ponder.[21] Or consider that quintessential of nervous disease, hysteria. Risse's work has shown that the actual experience at the Edinburgh Royal Infirmary belies the stereotype of hysteria as a class-specific behavioural phenomenon.[22] Nor does Cullen make it so in his formal writings: while insisting that it is most common in women between puberty and the age of thirty-five; and in unmarried or widowed than in married women; and is often associated with the menstrual period; he also held that it could occur in men, and that among women, it was commonest in those with 'the most robust and masculine constitutions'.[23] His epidemiology of hysteria was based on climate rather than innate characteristics of women. As he wrote,

> proper hysteric diseases . . . are more seldom met with in cold countries. Accordingly, instead of a cold bath, living in a cold air is a better method to obviate these disorders, the air here acting as a permanent cold. The common air of our climate is excellently adapted for hysteric patients; while living in warm rooms, over a fire, is sure to increase their complaints. For this reason it is, that in the hottest climates spasmodic distempers are more common and severe than in the more northern. The tetanus, the most violent of this class, is almost peculiar to the torrid zone; while in the same way in Europe, the hysteric disease, and, indeed, spasmodic complaints in general, are more severe in Spain and Italy than in France, Switzerland or England; and, as I am inclined to think, more so in England than with us. It is, I believe, common for a woman to threaten her husband with a fit in England, which I never knew or heard of here.[24]

Cold, it seems, had its uses. Much of this, of course was consistent with Enlightenment environmentalism, though it was also couched with Cullen's usual caution: 'I am inclined to think', 'I believe'.[25]

Equally important for present purposes are his references in the passage just quoted to tetanus and 'other spasmodic distempers'. In the remainder of this essay I shall examine how the breadth of Cullen's categories of nervous diseases – the neuroses – reflects certain fundamental aspects of the neurophysiology he expounded in the *Institutes*: how, more precisely, Cullen's neurophysiology was actually a neuromuscular physiology.

It is well known that the great Swiss polymath Albrecht von Haller made, on the basis of extensive experimentation, the distinction between two fundamental properties of animals: sensibility, which he associated with nerves; and irritability, which he identified as an inherent property of muscles. The consequence of sensibility was feeling; that of irritability was movement or contraction.[26] It is also well-known that Whytt could not accept Haller's distinction, preferring to conceptualize the operation throughout the body of an unconscious 'sentient principle', whose agency was the nervous system. The Haller-Whytt debate has been described by various historians and need not concern us here.[27]

While Cullen was not simply a slavish follower of Whytt, he was at one with his colleague in rejecting Haller's distinction between sensibility and irritability: for Cullen, there was no clear distinction between the nervous system and the muscles. At the very beginning of his *Institutes* he postulated a kind of functional hierarchy, consisting, in ascending order, of muscle, nerve, brain, will and sense. At first blush, it seems odd that he should place sense above will, but as he remarked, 'The will may be primary and independent, but . . . we can, for the most part, very clearly perceive that the will arises in consequence of sense. Unless I see you before me, or unless I at least imagine you present before me, I will not open my mouth to speak'.[28] Elsewhere, he remarked, 'Withdraw Sensation and the system falls asleep',[29] a wise injunction for lecturers.

But what of the muscles, those 'most remarkable organs'? There is, Cullen insisted, hardly any sort of motion, connected with any function, not performed by muscles, or muscular fibres; further, no muscular fibre lacks its connexion with nerves: destroy the nerve and you destroy the action of the muscles. The nervous system, in fact, he considered to consist of four parts, (1) what he called the 'medullary substance' in the cranium and vertebral cavity, i.e. the brain and spinal cord; (2) membraneous nerves which are continuous with the medullary substance; (3) sensory nerves which he conceived to be divested of their enveloping membrane and to serve as a series of windows to the outside world; and finally:

> (4) Certain extremities of the nerves so framed as to be capable of a peculiar contractility, and, in consequence of their situation and attachments, to be, by their contraction, capable of moving most of the solid and fluid parts of the body. These we name the MOVING EXTREMITIES of the nerves: they are commonly named MOVING or MUSCULAR FIBRES.[30]

This is a sweeping statement, and one which Cullen recognised as controversial, for as he admitted, anatomists had not shown that muscular fibres are a continuation of nerves, nor did most physiologists admit it: but, he gamely ventured, 'we now suppose it'.

I cannot here examine in any detail Cullen's discussion of the nature of muscular action, or his attempt to differentiate his own position from that of Haller or Whytt. He was himself no experimentalist, and most of his new experimental evidence was taken from the 1767 thesis of a student of his, Thomas Smith, entitled *De Actione Musculari*. Little is known of Smith except that he came from Staffordshire, and that he enrolled in a number of classes in Edinburgh between 1757 and 1767, being particularly fond of Cullen's chemistry classes.[31] It has been impossible to identify him with any certainty after 1767. What Smith showed, and Cullen incorporated, was that muscles could be stimulated to contract either by direct application of various mechanical or chemical means to muscle itself, or to its nerve; and that, when the muscle was no longer able to react, excitation of neither muscle nor its nerve was effective. They were thus functionally continuous and therefore, Cullen reasoned, part of the same system, i.e. the nervous system.

There is an irony here. William Cullen, reputedly one of the architects of the modern concept of nervous diseases, expounded a traditional and, by his time, outmoded view of the relationship between the nervous and the muscular systems. In insisting on their essential identity, Cullen harked back to the Greek world when tendons and sinews and nerves were ill-distinguished; when 'nervous' meant 'well strung; strong; vigorous';[32] back to a time when an etymologically related word we still use had other connotations. In Stephen Blancard's seventeenth-century medical dictionary, the first in English, we read under the definition for *Aponeurosis*: 'the End Tail or String of Muscles: 'tis call'd also a tendon. Chirurgeons take it falsely for a Nerve'.[33] Whether Cullen was conscious that in dropping the 'apo' from aponeurosis, one was left with the name of his new class of disease, I do not known. Possibly not, since the same Greek root lay behind both.

Whether Cullen was physiologically or anatomically justified in retaining this traditional formal connexion between muscle and nerves is beside the point: what it did for Cullen the clinician and nosologist was of great consequence, however, for it permitted him to broaden the class of diseases he called neuroses and to make literal sense of the traditional proposition that the principal functions of the nervous system are concerned with sense and motion: 'under the title of NEUROSIS [I comprehend] all those preternatural affections of sense and motion which are without pyrexia, as a part of the primary disease'.[34]

Two other points expounded in Cullen's *First Lines* need to be noticed before we can comprehend the variety of disorders he grouped together. First, he retained the traditional Galenic division of physiological functions into the vital, the natural and the animal, despite certain difficulties. For instance, the functions of the heart and lungs were commonly considered vital, but Cullen believed that the action of the heart is 'dependent on the energy of the brain', and neurological functions were classically identified with the animal ones. Second, he argued for the essential unity of all muscular fibres. One source of disagreement between Whytt and Haller had been over the fact that Haller's distinction between irritability and sensibility seemed to require rather different explanatory mechanisms to account for the actions of voluntary and involuntary muscles, a problem Whytt believed he had solved by referring everything back to the nervous system and its sentient principle. For Cullen, muscle contraction can occur as a result of the action of a nerve. This he called 'Nervous Power'. In addition, however, muscles possess in varying degrees, and, independently of their connexion with the other parts of the nervous system,[35] a power to contract. This was Haller's *vis insita*. Cullen named it the 'inherent power'.

While Cullen's compromise lacked the elegance of simplicity, it provided him with the physiological background for what was clearly for him the more congenial work of describing and classifying diseases. Now, I shall not poach on Professor Kendell's territory and examine Cullen's nosological work in detail. Nevertheless, two brief points need to be made about the class, neuroses. First, an appreciation of Cullen's views on the interconnexions between muscles and nerves helps us appreciate the logic behind what at first glance seems a smorgasbord of conditions which he defined as neuroses: why should cholera or diabetes be classed in the same group as more familiar 'nervous' disorders, such as hysteria, hypochondriasis and mania?[36] What is the connexion between dyspepsia and whooping cough? The answer, of course, is that each involves a disturbance of either sensation or motion. For instance, the apparently ragbag order of spasmodic afflictions neatly divides into three main divisions, spasms involving the animal functions and thereby voluntary muscles, such as epilepsy and tetanus; those involving the vital ones, such as palpitations of the heart and asthma; and those involving the natural ones, such as cholic and hysteria. At the other extreme, the loss of animal functions rates its own order, the comata, consisting of apoplexy and palsy; whereas those of the vital and natural functions are grouped together as *Adynamiae*, and include fainting, dyspepsia and hypochondriasis. The logic of his division required that both hysteria and hypochondriasis could be diagnosed in both sexes.

The second point should also be obvious: Cullen's category of the neuroses is not in any meaningful way exclusively psychiatric, or even neuropsychiatric in the modern sense. Even López Piñero, in his *Historical origins of the concept of neurosis*, has modernised Cullen, in looking almost exclusively at how his predecessors dealt with the two grand neuroses, hysteria and hypochondriasis, and in concentrating perhaps too much on Cullen's psychiatric followers.[37] To be sure, the ultimate legacy was undoubtedly psychiatric, but by stressing from the beginning only those portions of Cullen's category which still seem appropriate to our notion of the neurosis, López Piñero loses sight of the actual class which Cullen elaborated.

It was through a consideration of deranged motions of the stomach that Cullen justified at some length including dyspepsia among his neuroses. While admitting that the symptoms of dyspepsia – want of appetite, heartburn, stomach pains, vomiting – could be secondary to some other cause, such as ulcer or tumour, he believed that the symptoms more generally constituted a genus of disease to be further distinguished by their associated condition. No other organ except the brain, he held, had such a close connexion with the nervous system, and with no organ was the power of sympathy, or the *vis medicatrix naturae*, so apparent. Biliousness had been throughout the century a common fellow traveller in the cluster of nervous complaints: Cullen provided a physiological rationale.

It has often been remarked that Cullen was disappointed to have had to content himself for a while with teaching merely the Institutes of Medicine, instead of its practice. It is clear, however, that the two aspects of his work were related, just as it is equally apparent that his physiology was that of a clinician. He was not an experimentalist and derived his neuromuscular physiology from many sources, including Boerhaave, Hoffmann, Hales, Whytt, and Gaub as well as his student Thomas Smith. Whether his decision to view the muscles as part of the nervous system was necessary to enable him to lump disorders which earlier nosologists had split, is a hypothetical question. My own opinion is that it was, and that not for the first or last time in the history of medicine has a man who is most correctly seen as a traditionalist found himself in the role of innovator. This nervous Dr Cullen, it turns out, was something of a muscle man.

Acknowledgements

I am grateful for the efficient and knowledgeable help provided by Dr Michael Barfoot, Archivist of the Lothian Health Board. I also benefited from discussions with my colleagues Roy Porter and Chris Lawrence. My thanks also go to the President and Fellows of the Royal College of Physicians of Edinburgh for inviting me to participate in the Cullen Symposium, and for their warm hospitality during it. Betty Kingston and Sally Bragg have coped wonderfully with the vagaries of my handwriting. As always, the staff of the Wellcome Institute Library were cheerfully helpful. Research expenses have been provided by the Wellcome Trust.

Notes and references

1. J. Thomson, *An Account of the Life, Lectures, and Writings of William Cullen*, 2 vols (Edinburgh: William Blackwood and Sons, 1859), I: 25. Volume I was first published in 1832 and was reissued when the second volume was completed by William Thomson, who died in 1852, and David Craigie. Henceforth, I shall refer to it as Thomson, *Life*.

2. J. Thomson, ed., *The Works of William Cullen*, 2 vols (Edinburgh: William Blackwood and Sons, 1827), II: 330. Henceforth, Cullen, *Works*.

3. Quoted in J. Spillane, *The Doctrine of the Nerves* (Oxford: Oxford University Press, 1981), 138.

4. For general discussions of these issues, cf. W.F. Bynum, 'The Nervous Patient in Eighteenth and Nineteenth Century Britain: the Psychiatric Origins of British Neurology', in W.F. Bynum, R. Porter and M. Shepherd, eds., *The Anatomy of Madness*, 2 vols (London: Tavistock, 1985), 89–102; and R. Porter, 'Introduction' to facsimile reprint of George Cheyne's *The English Malady* (London: Tavistock/ Routledge, 1990).

5. Thomson, *Life*, I: 200; cf. I.A. Bowman, 'William Cullen (1710–1790) and the Primacy of the Nervous System' (Unpub. Ph.D. thesis, Indiana University, 1975).

6. E. Clarke, trans. and ed., *The Historical Development of Experimental Brain and Spinal Cord Physiology before Flourens*, by M. Neuberger (Baltimore: Johns Hopkins University Press, 1981).

7. E. Clarke and C.D. O'Malley, *The Human Brain and Spinal Cord* (Los Angeles: University of California Press, 1968).

8. E. Clarke and L.S. Jacyna, *Nineteenth-Century Origins of Neuroscientific Concepts* (Los Angeles: University of California Press, 1987).

9. Spillane, *op. cit.* (note 3).

10. F.H. Garrison, *An Introduction to the History of Medicine*, 4th ed., (Philadelphia: W.B. Saunders Company, 1929), 358.

11. C. Lawrence, 'The Nervous System and Society in the Scottish Enlightenment', in B. Barnes and S. Shapin, eds., *Natural Order* (Beverley Hills, California: Sage Publications, 1979), 19–40.

12. C. Lawrence, 'Medicine as Culture: Edinburgh and the Scottish Enlightenment' (Unpub. Ph.D. thesis, University of London, 1984).

13. Cullen, *Works*, I: 19.

14. In addition to the works of Lawrence (notes 11, 12), cf. J.P. Wright, 'Metaphysics and Physiology: Mind, Body, and the Animal Economy in Eighteenth-Century Scotland', *Oxford Studies in the History of Philosophy* (1990), I: 251–301; and M. Barfoot, 'James Gregory (1753–1821) and Scottish Scientific Metaphysics, 1750–1800' (Unpub. Ph.D. thesis, Edinburgh University, 1983), esp. ch. 5.

15. J. Todd, *Sensibility* (London: Methuen, 1986), surveys this development.

16. Quoted in R. Porter, *Mind-Forg'd Manacles: A History of Madness in England from the Restoration to the Regency* (London: Athlone, 1987), 105. The relationship between 'spirits', and the physiology of 'nerves' is complicated: cf. G.S. Rousseau, 'Nerves, Spirits and Fibres: Towards Defining the Origins of Sensibility; With a Postscript', *The Blue Guitar* (1976), II: 125–53; *idem*, 'Psychology' in G.S. Rousseau and R. Porter, eds., *The Ferment of Knowledge* (Cambridge: Cambridge University Press, 1980), 143–210.

17. The whole passage from Adair's *Medical Cautions, for the Consideration of Invalids* (1786) is quoted in R. Hunter and I. MacAlpine, *Three Hundred Years of Psychiatry* (Oxford: Oxford University Press, 1963), 489–90.

18. R. Hunter and I. Macalpine, *George III and the Mad-Business* (London: Allen Lane, 1969), 288.

19. Cullen, *Works*, II: 465.

20. There is an important unpublished essay 'On the Effects of Custom on the Organs of Sensation' in the Cullen Manuscripts (Box 4, no. 12) in the University of Glasgow Library. I am indebted to Dr Michael Barfoot for the reference, and to the Librarian of Glasgow University for supplying me with a xerox copy.

21. Above, note 2. For a recent evaluation of John Brown and his influence, cf. W.F. Bynum and R. Porter, eds., *Brunonianism in Britain and Europe, Medical History*, Supplement No. 8, 1988.

22. G.B. Risse, *Hospital Life in Enlightenment Scotland* (Cambridge: Cambridge University Press, 1986); *idem*, 'Hysteria at the Edinburgh Infirmary; the Construction and Treatment of a Disease, 1770–1800', *Medical History*, 32 (1988), 1–22.

23. Cullen, *Works*, II: 495.

24. *Ibid.*, 505–6.

25. There is a good discussion of eighteenth-century environmentalism in C.J. Glacken, *Traces on the Rhodian Shore* (Los Angeles: University of California Press, 1967), chs. 12–13.

26. The 1755 English translation of Haller's *De Partibus Corporis Humani Sensibilibus et Irritabilibus* was reprinted, with a useful introduction by O. Temkin, in *Bulletin of the History of Medicine*, 4 (1936), 651–99.

27. E.g. R.K. French, *Robert Whytt, the Soul and Medicine* (London: Wellcome Institute, 1969).

28. Cullen, *Works*, I: 14ff; cf. Thomson, *Life*, I: 284ff.

29. R. Stott, 'Health and Virtue, or How to Keep Out of Harm's Way: Lectures on Pathology and Therapeutics by William Cullen, M.D. c.1770', *Medical History*, *31* (1987), 123–42, on 135.

30. Cullen, *works*, I: 15–16.

31. I owe this information to Michael Barfoot, who has also very kindly supplied me with a xerox of Smith's thesis, which is of more than ordinary interest. I hope to examine it more fully at a later date.

32. This is the first (and preferred) definition of 'Nervous' in Samuel Johnson, *A Dictionary of the English Language*, 2 vols (London: W. Strahan, 1755).

33. Stephen Blancard, *The Physical Dictionary*, 6th ed. (London: Sam. Crouch, 1715). Earlier editions have the same definition.

34. Cullen, *Works*, II: 330.

35. *Ibid.*, I: 64. My emphasis.

36. Cullen's 'cholera' was of course the milder gastro-intestinal disease, rather than the 'Asian' cholera which preoccupied doctors in the ninetenth century.

37. J.M. López Piñero, *Historical Origins of the Concept of Neurosis*, trans. D. Berrios (Cambridge: Cambridge University Press, 1983).

6

General practice in Hamilton
Baillie Cullen – country doctor extraordinaire

E. GRAHAM BUCKLEY

When the President invited me to contribute to this Symposium my first re-action was to decline. What did I know about Cullen, about eighteenth-century medicine and, in particular, about general practice in that century? The answer was and is precious little. My qualification is that I am a general practitioner and can claim kinship with Cullen in that I practice very near to where he is buried in Kirknewton and that I have received my medical education in the Medical Faculty and in the clinical tradition which he was so instrumental in creating.

Starting from a position of ignorance has some advantage. All that I have read about Cullen and medicine in the eighteenth century has been fresh and vivid. My holiday reading has never been so enjoyable. William Cullen was clearly a man who inspired loyalty and trust. From his own writings he emerges as a diligent, observant, modest and amiable man who possessed a great warmth and charm. In these respects he represents the best of the Age of Reason. Enough of eulogies and generalities, what of general practice, what of Cullen as a general practitioner and what of Hamilton?

The first point to make is that in his own terms he was a country doctor in Hamilton. The term general practitioner was not used until after his death. This is more than a semantic distinction. In the eighteenth century doctors, using that term in a very wide sense, became relevant and available for the first time to the majority of the populace. Most of the regular doctors were surgeon apothecaries. Cullen was typical of the men who wished to become doctors at the beginning of the eighteenth century and typical initially in the route which he chose. The qualities which he brought to his calling helped to transform a trade into a profession.

Apprenticeship

Cullen's father was factor to the Duke of Hamilton and had a small estate himself. He also acted as a writer or lawyer in Hamilton. The records at the Society of Apothecaries in England show that two-thirds of apprentices were the sons of doctors, clergy or landed gentry. Records of apprentices in Bristol show a similar picture.

Cullen was a pupil at Hamilton Grammar School, where he 'was particularly distinguished by the liveliness of his manner, by an uncommon quickness of apprehension, and by a most retentive memory'. After leaving the school, Cullen spent time attending classes at Glasgow University before being apprenticed to Mr Paisley, a surgeon and apothecary in the city. Records from England show that apprentices could pay anything from £0–£250 per year for the privilege of working from 7am to 7pm making up the potions and draughts for patients as well as looking after the shop whilst the apothecary was out on his visits.

At the age of nineteen Cullen left the apothecary's shop in Glasgow and travelled to London seeking to become a ship's surgeon. This was an excellent way of acquiring practical experience in treating sailors suffering from a wide range of medical and surgical disorders. Because the ship's surgeon was a paid appointment and because of the excellent experience which it afforded, competition for the post was intense. The fact that Captain Cleland was a cousin cannot have done his chances any harm. He joined Captain Cleland for a nine-month tour of duty to the West Indies.

I could not find any account from Cullen himself about his experience as a ship's surgeon but others have written of the horrors of attempting to perform amputations on board ship and the tropical and deficiency diseases encountered.

Returning from the West Indies, Cullen worked as an assistant to an apothecary in London for a period of eighteen months. Captain Cleland must have been greatly impressed by his ability as a doctor for he then asked Cullen to return to Scotland to look after his ailing son in Auchinlea, near Shotts.

In 1733 he inherited a small legacy and this enabled him to pursue his studies by matriculating in the University of Edinburgh. It was during his time at the University that a student society was founded which later became the Royal Medical Society. Of the many student societies which were formed at that time, it is the one which has prospered to the present day and I am looking forward to the meeting later this evening in the modern premises of the Society. The foundation of the Royal Medical Society is evidence of the energy and independence shown by students in the medical faculty in the early eighteenth century.

General practice in Hamilton

After two years at Edinburgh University, and still aged only twenty-six years, Cullen returned to Hamilton where he stayed and prospered in general practice for the next eight years. What kind of work did he do? His account books give an interesting insight into his work for the household of the Duke of Hamilton. The ledgers show the importance of the livestock and the chaotic nature of therapeutics at that time. The account books show the importance of dispensing as the method by which doctors charged for their services. Scotland fortunately avoided the major conflicts which arose in London between physicians and apothecaries. This conflict centred on apothecaries being able to charge for dispensing but not for visits whereas physicians charged for visits but not for dispensing.

It is apparent from his account books that Cullen was content to dispense drugs in bulk for the animals, but medicines for the family were dispensed in very small amounts.

Cullen's work as a general practitioner demonstrates in a very stark way the clinical paradox highlighted by Richard Asher:

> clinicians need to give patients confidence in the outcome of therapeutic interventions;
>
> clinicians need to remain sceptical about the efficacy of their interventions

There is no doubt that Cullen did inspire great confidence. The Duke of Hamilton did not wish him to leave and asked Cullen to accompany him on his visits to Arran and south of the border. The townspeople of Hamilton elected him Chief Magistrate or Provost on two occasions. Later in his life when requests for his medical opinion were received from all over Europe, his detailed, but down to earth, advice carried conviction and authority. At the same time his lectures and experiments indicate that he was aware of the inadequate evidence for the efficacy of conventional treatments and that errors in diagnosis were frequently exposed in the dissecting room.

What were the common clinical problems he would encounter in general practice in Hamilton? First and foremost fevers, which were categorised as continued, intermittent, remittent, and eruptive. The fever itself was thought to be a unifying aspect of a whole range of different diseases. Cullen, with his orderly mind, attempted to define and discriminate between different types of disease. Most of the fevers were due to infections and it is hard in the modern era to appreciate the fear and risk associated with these infections. Typhus and smallpox were still common in Scotland at that time. Many medical men, as well as patients, died of typhus which often wiped out whole medical families.

Next to the fevers were diarrhoeal diseases. Among the chronic diseases arthritis and gout were recognised but perhaps the most distressing was the phthisis seen in children and young adults. Apart from this condition it is unlikely that Cullen saw many children. Ailments in children were usually looked after by irregular practitioners using traditional and folk remedies.

The greatest similarity between general practice in the eighteenth century and modern practice would be in the management of minor surgical and obstetric problems. Before the eighteenth century doctors were not involved in midwifery, but Smellie in Lanark who became a pioneer in British obstetrics corresponded with Cullen and, as the century advanced, surgeon-apothecaries added the skills and title of 'man midwife' to their advertisements.

Cullen himself appears not to have enjoyed the practical aspects of a surgeon's work and avoided setting limbs, incising abscesses etc. by subcontracting this work to another surgeon apothecary.

Although Cullen, both in Hamilton and on a larger scale later in Edinburgh, was very successful, he did not die a rich man. It is very difficult to estimate his likely income. Little work has been done on the income of doctors in Scotland in the eighteenth century. From his account books his income from the Duke of Hamilton appears to have been in the region of £30–£60 per annum. These were probably pounds English rather than pounds Scots. He would probably charge for visits as well as dispensing, and from his position in the town it is likely that he earned more than a lawyer and more than the average farmer. Evidence from England indicates that income could be anything from £100 to £1,000 per annum and that Scottish doctors were generally regarded as being less well off. Again from England there are examples of doctors who earned the majority of their income from attending single households. Because of the rise in the number of practitioners, it is likely that income declined between 1750 and 1850.

I am aware that I have touched upon only some of the characteristics of general practice and general practitioners in the 1730s to 1740s. My admiration for Cullen has grown with my increasing knowledge of him. Perhaps the most impressive thing about this man is that in one year, 1740, he managed to run a busy practice, to take his Doctor of Medicine degree in the University of Glasgow and to woo his bride. Having successfully achieved all that, his subsequent success could have been expected. To the rest of the world he may be remembered as Professor Cullen of the Medical Faculty of Edinburgh University but I shall remember him as Baillie Cullen of Hamilton.

Acknowledgement

I wish to thank Dr Irvine Loudon for his help in preparing this paper.

Further reading

Loudon, I., *Medical care and the general practitioner 1750–1850*, Oxford: Clarendon Press, 1987.

7

William Cullen and dietetics

R. PASSMORE

We have two sources of information about Cullen's views on dietetics. These are the letters written to patients or their doctors and his lectures given to medical students. Cullen had a large consultant practice; patients or their doctors from all over Scotland and some from England, Europe and North America sought his advice. More than 2,000 of his letters to patients or their doctors were bound and are now in the College library. A few of these are in Cullen's own hand, but most were made by ammanuenses. After 1780 the copies of his letters were made with James Watt's duplicating machine (pp. 69–71). Most of the letters contain advice about diet, what the patient should eat. This is nearly always followed by advice on what exercise to take and what clothing to wear (Cullen was very aware of the vagaries of the Scottish climate), on hours of sleep and, when practical, on a change of air by a visit to a spa or a sea voyage. He thus followed Hippocrates and other classical Greek writers in recommending a διαιτα or way of living, which he translated as a regimen. He restricted the use of the word diet to a person's regular foods, as we do today.

Cullen included in his lectures to students on materia medica a large section on aliments. These lectures were given only once in the 1760–1 session but were greatly appreciated. So much so that the students prepared a transcript of them and this was published in London in 1772 without Cullen's knowledge. He was naturally very upset (pp. 92–3), especially as it contained numerous minor errors. However he allowed an amended version to be issued. As he was then engaged in writing other books, he did not get down to preparing his own version for many years. In 1789, the year before his death, his *Treatise of the Materia Medica* in two volumes was published. A section entitled *Of Aliments* is 214 pages long and forms just over half of volume I.

Cullen's practice and teaching on dietetics was based on his clinical experience and was thus almost entirely empirical. Neither the chemistry nor the physiology that he taught to large classes in Glasgow and Edinburgh universities provided significant material for a scientific background to dietetics. Indeed the science of nutrition is often stated to have originated from the work of Lavoisier in Paris in the last decade of the eighteenth century and immediately after Cullen's death. Despite the lack of a scientific background, most of the dietetic advice that he gave to his patients would now be considered sound and sensible medical practice. As it was given clearly, in detail and with authority but without confusing and possibly uncertain science, patients' compliance with advice might have been better than it is today.

Consultation letters

A letter to the Earl of Panmure's doctor is reproduced as an example of Cullen's style (RCPE Cullen MS 30, vol. 14, letter 15 June 1781). It emphasises the greater importance that he gave in the management of most diseases to advising a patient on a regimen, including a diet, than to prescribing medicines.

> After considering attentively the history of his Lordship's former and present complaints we are of the opinion that they have been very entirely rheumatic . . .
>
> His Lordship should now go to the country as soon as possible and when there should be as much in the fresh air as the weather and other circumstances will allow. He may walk out very often but exercise in this way should always be very moderate and never go the degree of being in the least heated or fatigued by it . . . In every situation the utmost care is to be taken to avoid cold and therefore his Lordship should not lay off his flannel waistcoat perhaps at any time and at least while any degree of pain or stiffness remains in any part of his body.
>
> By air and gentle exercise it is to be hoped that every ailment will be dissipated but it will also be proper at the same time to give attention to diet.
>
> Every morning his Lordship may take a draught or two of fresh drawn cow milk whey so that upon the whole about an English pint is taken. Half a pint may be taken pretty early and his Lordship may sleep after it . . .
>
> His Lordship's ordinary breakfast of tea and bread may be taken but tea in the least strong we think very improper and if his Lordship could in place of it take a basin of new milk we think it may be useful in the present state of things.
>
> At dinner his Lordship may take soup and a bit of any plain light meat he likes best but till everything rheumatic is entirely gone we would wish to avoid a full meal of meat and would always have a great part of it made up with pudding and vegetables.
>
> For ordinary drink we think sherry diluted with a good deal of water will be best and that all sort of malt liquors should be

avoided. Every day at dinner his Lordship may take two or three glasses of claret or of white wine and water but we need not say to his Lordship that the quantity of either be very moderate.

A dish of coffee in the afternoon if not very strong we think very allowable.

At supper for some time we think his Lordship should hardly take any solid food and that some kind of milk, meat or vegetables are the most proper.

By air, exercise and the above regimen we expect that his Lordship will get perfectly well and we have but one medicine to propose to assist in the business. It is a balsamic Tincture prescribed on a paper. [Here follow details of dosage]

Edinburgh   WILLIAM CULLEN
    15 June 1781

As a second example the dietetic advice in a letter for Mr Charles Abercrombie who was diagnosed as having nervous dyspepsia is given (RCPE Cullen MS 30, vol. 3, letter 3 August 1771).

He must always keep his stomach light and never make a full meal. He may take a bit of any plain meat every day at dinner but it should be a little only and make it up with broth, pudding and even vegetables. If he chooses these only which are young and tender he will bear them very well and his blood would be spoiled by his avoiding them altogether. He may continue to take fruits while he finds that his stomach agrees with them but he must avoid excess in raw fruit. The strawberries and gooseberries are pretty safe, but cherries and other stone fruits are most dangerous, and ripe pears are safer than apples.

In taking meat he must avoid all fat and heavy [sic], all fryed and baked. The light white fish as haddock, whiting, codling or flounder boiled and taken with very little butter will probably agree with him, but he must not take them often, nor at the same time as flesh.

For breakfast I think there is nothing better than cocoa, tea or very weak chocolate. Bohea or green tea are both bad for him and coffee is little better. For supper he should always take milk with bread or some kind of grain, and I think he should always take a little supper as it is much better to divide his meals than to take much at any one.

For ordinary drink toast water is certainly the best, and that without any addition, but if he requires it with some taste he may add a little strong wine to it as Madeira, sherry or red port. For strong drink he should take very little of any kind, but if there is occasion for it the strong wines just now mentioned taken always with a little water are safest.

Browsing through these hundreds of letters, I have been struck by the sameness of the dietetic advice given in almost all of them. Yet each letter is different and tailored to the circumstances of the patient. Cullen took care to prescribe in detail for each patient; he would have had little use for printed diet sheets.

Throughout the letters the emphasis is on moderation, but nowhere is moderation defined. A patient is never asked to weigh out a portion of food and it is left to his or her judgement to decide what is moderate. Also although many of his prosperous patients would have been overweight, none of them were asked to weigh themselves.

Cullen emphasises that it is best to spread the food intake through three meals. In the eighteenth century the main meal in the home of all classes was dinner, which was usually eaten at about 2 o'clock. However among the professional classes it was often postponed until 4 o'clock or even later to enable the meal to be eaten after the day's work was ended. Such dinners, we know, were often heavy. Many of Cullen's patients were advised to curtail their intake of meat at dinner and only to eat meat once a day.

Most of the letters give advice about appropriate physical exercise but none of those read give warnings about the dangers arising from tobacco. During Cullen's life many Glasgow merchants made fortunes out of importing tobacco from Virginia, but most of this was then exported to countries on the European continent. In Scotland inhaling snuff became fashionable among men in the eighteenth century who also smoked cigars and sometimes pipes. Despite the warnings given in the previous century by James VI on the health hazards of tobacco, smoking was not recognised as a cause of disease and tobacco is not mentioned in William Buchan's *Domestic Medicine*.

Of Aliments is the title of part I of Cullen's *A Treatise of the Materia Medica* which forms nearly a quarter of the two volumes. The treatise was his last book written when he was over seventy years of age, but it follows in general his lectures given over twenty years previously, which were taken down by students and published without his knowledge (p. 92). The first section on aliments in general gives an account of what we now call the science of nutrition. It is of necessity brief, only 21 pages. The remainder of the part contains a detailed description of all the foods commonly eaten in Europe and North America, and also of many eaten only occasionally or in a local community, and of those foods of tropical origin which were currently available. The place of each of these foods in dietetic practice is discussed.

Of aliments in general

The breakdown of foods into soluble products and the disposal of these in the body – the physiology of nutrition – and the chemical nature of foods are described.

The solid matter in foods is converted into a fluid form 'by the powers of the animal economy'.

The fluids of the body appear to be of many different kinds; but we can particularly distinguish those that are pretty constantly in the course of the circulation, which we call the *common mass*, from those found in other vessels than those concerned in the circulation. These, however, being all of them, as we presume, drawn from the common mass and therefore originally of the same matter, only somewhat changed by the secretory organs through which these pass . . . (p. 219)

A considerable part of the common mass is what we have named gluten or coaguable lymph. This I consider the chief part of the mass, because I suppose it to be the part of it which gives the matter of the solids, or the permanent constituent parts of the body, and which, from the beginning to the end of life, are constantly receiving a further accretion and increase. (p. 219) When this animal mixt is fully formed, it does not long remain stationary in that condition, but seems to be constantly, although perhaps slowly, proceeding to a putrid or putrescent stage. (p. 220). In this progress, as in other processes of putrefaction, we find the mild and perfectly neutral substance changed into a saline state of the ammoniacal kind. (p. 220) The animal fluid is considerably different in its qualities from the vegetable matter of which it is often entirely formed that this vegetable matter, after it has been taken into the body, is thus changed by the peculiar powers of the animal economy (p. 220) which it must be acknowledged is by no means clearly or fully understood. (p. 224)

Cullen pointed out that all aliments were ultimately derived from vegetable matter since this was the source, direct or indirect, of foods derived from animals. Not all vegetable matter was an alimentary matter and certain vegetables contained more of this than others. He concluded that

it appears that the matter of vegetables, whether in the whole or in the different parts of them, fitted to form the animal fluid, is an acid, a sugar and an oil (p. 227).

Acid

That this is a part of the common matter of vegetables which proves alimentary will be readily admitted, because it appears in the whole substance of many of our foods, and particularly is frequently very copious in vegetable fruits. In these, indeed, it is commonly combined with more or less of sugar; but from what happens in the progress of the maturation of fruits, which is often the change of an acid into a saccharine matter, it is to be presumed that an acid enters largely into the composition of sugar, and is thereby, as will be shown hereafter, a necessary ingredient in the composition of the animal fluid (p. 227).

Vegetables undergo fermentation with the production of acid and whenever a vegetable aliment is taken into the stomach an acid is always more or less evolved. At the same time it must be allowed, that as in the further progress of the aliment this acid disappears very entirely without being ever again evident in the mass of blood; so its having been entered into the composition of the animal fluid can hardly be doubted (p. 227).

As acids in vegetable aliments slowed down advances to the putrid state in animal fluids, Cullen supported the view that scurvy was a disease in which putrescence of these fluids had proceeded too far. It might perhaps be cured by every kind of acescent aliment, but especially by those in a state in nature, such as lemons or by vegetables converted by art into an acid state, as in sauerkraut. He had reason to believe that fossil (inorganic) acids did not enter into the composition of animal fluids. They readily passed unchanged into the excretions and did not cure scurvy. What may happen to phosphoric acid 'we do not very certainly know'. 'What notice is to be taken of the aerial or mephitic acid (CO_2), I am not well determined to say.' (p. 229)

Sugar

Cullen had doubts as to whether sugar in the pure state was alimentary, but it might be, since negresses on the sugar plantations grew plump and fat when they took a great deal of cane-juice. However;

a great proportion of sugar is contained in all farinaceous matter . . . being evolved by their germination or malting (p. 230). Farinaceous feeds are of all other vegetable matters the most powerful and nourishing to men, as well as domestic animals; and hence the *Farina Alibilis* of Dr Haller (the Swiss physiologist). This nutritious quality he imputes to a mucilageous or gelatinous matter which appears in them upon their being diffused in water. This, he thinks, may be the basis of its nutritive quality. This vegetable mucilage consists for the greater part of sugar. We allow it, however, to be also probable, that farina consists of another matter, which may be supposed to give the whole its gelatinous appearance in solution, and probably also to render the whole a more proper, complete and powerful nourishment to the human body. This other ingredient of farina is probably an oil (p. 231).

Oil

Oils, whether taken into the body as part of the vegetable foods or in a

pure form after expression from vegetable matter is a fundamental part
of the human aliment. Four considerations support this statement.

> 1st, Oil, both from vegetable and animal substances, is daily taken
> in as part of the diet of all nations, and often in large quantity
> without increasing obesity . . . It is not separate from other fluids of
> the alimentary canal but is very accurately diffused in the chyle;
> which may be considered a step towards a more intimate mixture
> (p. 233).
> 2dly, That such a mixture takes place is very probable from this that
> no chyle appears in the left ventricle of the heart. 3rdly, not only no
> chyle but neither does any oil ever appear in the mass of the blood,
> nor ever in any part of the human body, till it appears in the cellular
> or adipose membrane, into which it is probably brought by a
> peculiar secretion (p. 233).
> A fourth consideration that leads to suppose the oil taken in is often
> copiously laid up in the adipose membrane of healthy animals, is
> again, upon various occasions, absorbed and taken into the course
> of the circulation. Some of these occasions are manifestly those
> states in which a great degree of acrimony prevails in the mass of
> blood, as in scorbutic, syphilitic, hectic and other such cases; and
> while it is highly probable that the purpose of such absorption is by
> the oil to cover the acrimony of the animal fluid, it must prove at
> the same time that this admits of an intimate mixture with the oil
> (p. 234).

After a page discussing whether gum arabic is an alimentary, the
conclusion is reached that

> the vegetable matters affording aliment are acid, sugar, and oil,
> which in diet may be taken in, sometimes in their pure state; but
> . . . more commonly and perhaps more properly, be taken in in a
> combined state; and in the latter case, either as they are combined
> in vegetable substances by nature, or as they are joined together by
> the cook in the preparations of diet (p. 236).

Then follows a caveat. The Italian, Beccaria, is quoted as having
discovered in wheat and other flours a substance that is coagulable and
nourishing. This matter 'in its nature approaches more nearly to the
nature of animal substance than any other part of vegetable matter we
know of' (p. 236). But this discovery does not invalidate the conclusion
that the chief part of vegetable aliment is made up of acid, sugar and oil.

The section ends with a brief discussion of 'the power of the gastric
menstruum' on different substances. Some foods are more easily
solubilised than others, and 'as the arts of cookery render the texture of
aliments more tender, it renders them in proportion more soluble in the
stomach' (p. 238). Men liable to rumination and eructation provide

evidence that the solubilities of foods depends on many different circumstances.

Of particular aliments

This long and detailed catalogue gives accounts of the origins of foods in nature and, when applicable, methods of processing and cooking. Tenderness is frequently mentioned as this is associated with solubility in the gastric menstruum and so with digestibility.

Some preparations valuable in diets for invalids are described, for instance a form of whey.

> This dish, during the whole of the summer, in Scotland, is often used by the middling rank of people and is well known at Edinburgh under the name of Corstophin Cream, and as denominated from the neighbouring village, in which it is especially prepared; it is brought to market in all the considerable towns of Scotland. It is an aliment tolerably nourishing; and by the quantity of acid still retained in it is moderately, but gratefully, acid and cooling. I have frequently prescribed it to phthisical patients; and neither in these, nor in any other persons, have I ever known any disorders of the stomach or the intestines arising from the free use of it (p. 352).

Some new foods are described, for instance kohlrabi.

> I have become acquainted with a species of Brassica, *Brassica Gongylodes*, which, till I had raised it in my own garden, was not, as far as I can learn, known or produced in Britain. It is distinguished by its having on the upper part of its stalk a swelled part or spheroidical tuber, which within a firm cortical part is formed of a substance of the same nature with that which forms the medullary part in the stalks of cabbage and other kinds of colewort. This medullary part, when freed from its rind, and very well boiled, is of a tender and sweet substance, and certainly considerably nourishing, and appears to me to be less flatulent than the cabbage (p. 262).

Sometimes medicinal folklore is demolished.

> If the large annual use of strawberries could preserve from the gout, we should seldom find the inhabitants of Edinburgh inflicted with that disease; but though they use that supposed preservative very largely, we find them as often and as severely affected with the gout as the inhabitants of other places who do not use the same (p. 252).

What we now know as food allergy is described:

> Digestion is a mysterious business, which we do not in all its circumstances, well understand; and therefore we cannot at all explain the singular fact of the white of egg even in very small

quantity, whether in its liquid or coagulated state, proving constantly the occasion of much sickness in the stomach of certain persons, while in the most part of other men it is an agreeable and readily digested food (p. 383).

I have known several instances of persons who could not take even a small quantity of lobster or crab without being affected soon after with a violent colic, and sometimes with the same efflorescence on the skin which, as we said above, often happens from eating salmon or herrings. In both cases, I believe it happens from the idiosyncracy of particular persons; and how difficult that is to be explained, will appear from what we said above on the subject of Eggs (p. 393).

The places of milk, meats and alcoholic beverages in our diets arouse contentions today. In the eighteenth century they were likewise of interest, but perhaps less contentious, and Cullen has much to say about each of them.

Milk

Milk is described as 'a homogenous liquor, composed of an oil, a coagulable and a watery matter; vulgarly known under the names Cream, Curd and Whey' (p. 306). The domestic arts of separating these are given in some detail and especially that of cheese-making and the use of 'runnet'. That these component parts are present in different proportions in milks from various species of mammals is stated but no quantitative data are given. The very limited knowledge of their chemistry is discussed. Whey contains

a genuine sugar and differs from that of the sugar cane only by it sharing some of the oily or caseous parts of milk adhering to it, but from which it may, by repeated solutions and crystallizations, be entirely freed, and thereby be brought to the same degree of purity as any other sugar (p. 317).

This sugar can be fermented and

in time produces a considerable amount of acid, probably of a peculiar kind; though so far as I yet know, it has not been chemically examined (p. 318).

The coagulable part of milk is very much of the nature of animal substances; and if we shall adopt the common opinion, that milk is especially formed of the chyle or newly taken-in aliment, we shall readily perceive that this must be always blended with the lymph which it meets with in its passage through the lacteals and thoracic duct (p. 315).

Lactation

The physiology of lactation is discussed. Cullen argued that the common opinion that chyle, without being mixed with the blood, is carried directly to the mammae and appears there in the form of milk was wrong. Chyle enters the subclavian vein slowly and in small quantities and it would be impossible for it to appear in an artery as a separate mass.

> We shall find it much more probable that milk is produced in the mammae of females by the peculiar, though mysterious, powers of secretion . . .
> But although milk be not the same fluid which passed from the thoracic duct into the subclavian vein, there are many arguments which lead us to suppose that the matter of milk is chiefly afforded by the matter of the chyle, or of the alimentary matter last taken in (p. 322).

The question of what is a suitable diet for a nursing mother follows. This was much discussed at the time as many women moving in society handed their newborn infants over to wet-nurses to suckle. Cullen states that for a good output of milk, a nurse depends more on the quantity of liquid drunk than on the solid food. A nurse who has been for a time free of thirst may, as soon as an infant begins to suckle, have a strong desire to drink. Although women who can afford to do so commonly employ a mixed diet of animal and vegetable matter, there is no necessity for a nursing woman to take animal food.

> Supposing the quantity of liquid to be the same, nurses living entirely, or for the greater part, upon vegetable aliment, afford a greater quantity of milk, and of more proper quality, than nurses living upon much animal food. This I venture to assert from the experience of fifty years; during which time I have known innumerable instances of the healthiest children reared upon the milk of nurses living entirely upon vegetable aliments; and I have known many instances of children becoming diseased by their being fed by the milk of nurses who had changed their diet from being entirely vegetable to the taking of a quantity of animal food (p. 334).

A further reading for avoiding animal foods is given.

> It appears to me, that in nurses, for a certain length of time, the determination of the blood to the uterus and ovaria is suspended; so that during that time neither menstruation nor conception take place. We know, notwithstanding, that in some nurses both these states occur; and I am persuaded that they most readily take place in habits naturally plethoric, or rendered so by the large use of animal food. It is, however, generally and probably upon observation judged that both menstruation and conception are always incompatible with the proper condition of a nurse; and therefore to

avoid these inconveniences, it seems proper for nurses to avoid animal food altogether, or at least to take it sparingly (p. 336).

Cullen's suggestion that meat in the diet has an effect on female reproductory function has never, as far as I know, been followed up.

Cullen allays concern on two matters. First he has not known of a child affected by purgatives given to nurses. Secondly

Many nurses take in considerable quantities of intoxicating liquor and are themselves intoxicated by it; but I have not known any instances of the intoxicating power being communicated to their infants.

Paediatricians today are, of course, much more cautious in their advice on the use of drugs and alcohol by nursing mothers.

Infant feeding

While milk is judged to be the proper nourishment of newborn animals, there can hardly be a doubt, that to every newborn animal the milk best adapted to it must be that of the species it belongs to, and consequently that of the mother who had immediately produced it . . . How long this nourishment is the best adapted to infants, it is difficult to determine; but the very purpose of multiplying the species shows that nature has set some limits to it. So far as we can trust our observations on the human species, we find inconveniences from either too long or too short nursing: and it appears to me that either less than seven, or more than eleven, months is generally hurtful . . . From some accidental circumstances this measure may be safely varied; but what are the circumstances of the infant's condition that require it to be varied more or less, has not, that I know of, been properly ascertained . . . but I am persuaded that too long nursing contributes to increasing the disposition to rickets . . . How soon is it proper to employ an aliment of another kind? The very early introduction of vegetable aliment is improper; and we are persuaded that it cannot be introduced with safety for some months after the birth; but for how long precisely we dare not determine. From my own observations [Cullen had eight children], I am led to think that hardly in any case it should be introduced until five months are past; even after that period, it should be increased by degrees . . . so that at the time of weaning no considerable change may be made (pp. 330–31).

That some infants do not digest properly even their mother's milk may be due either to the state of the milk or to the state of the child's stomach. This is discussed at some length but not very helpfully and it is concluded that 'it must be left to skilful practitioners to judge of the causes in particular cases, and to direct their practice accordingly'.

Milk in diets for the healthy

Cullen's teaching was based on many years of careful observation. He knew empirically that in general milk and milk products were beneficial both in sickness and in health but that in some healthy people and in certain diseases they were not well tolerated. To explain these differences as far as possible he used the science of his day but, since the concept of energy had not been developed and protein had not been identified as a distinct nutrient, his explanations could not have helped his students much. Milk was 'of an intermediate nature between the entirely vegetable and entirely animal aliments'. Thus as its sugar was fermentable, it was acescent, but the caseous or coagulable part had, like all animal foods, a tendency to putrescence and so was potentially alkalescent.

> At every period of life . . . there can be little doubt of cows' milk being a sufficiently fit nourishment; but it may be more or less so at different periods. The younger children are . . . it seems to be the more fit . . . As it is doubtful if the human œconomy can be properly supported by vegetable aliment alone; so milk, as affording a portion of alkalescent matter, will be properly joined with it: and we known instances of a numerous people who are sustained in a condition fit for all the functions of life by milk and vegetable matter alone. There can be no doubt, therefore, of the propriety of rearing children in the same manner. I believe it is hardly ever necessary to give children under the age of puberty any quantity of animal food.

> We are indeed of the opinion that a certain proportion of animal food is intended by nature . . . and in cold climates, at the period of life when men are to be engaged in the laborious business of life, that animal food is then especially proper, and perhaps necessary, while at the same time that milk may be less sufficient for the purpose.

> How long this state may continue, I dare not determine; but whenever the powers and vigour of life begin to decline, we are persuaded that the alkalescent state of the fluids is always increasing as life advances; so the more this happens, we are inclined to think that the more plentiful use of milk and vegetables may be again introduced (p. 338).

Milk in diets for invalids

Milk is a restorative medicine. It can be used in all cases of emaciation and debility where the digestive organs are not affected.

Milk may 'moderate and perhaps cure' phthisis pulmonalis. This disease 'never discovers its peculiar symptoms without discovering at the same time a phlogistic diathesis in the whole system'. This term was used by Cullen for what we now call a general inflammatory response. 'As milk affords a less quantity of gluten, and a less alkalescent fluid, than any animal food; so it must be of service in obviating a phlogistic diathesis'. In this respect cows' milk may be less effective than that of non-ruminent animals such as asses and mares. A common opinion was that woman's milk was the best for this purpose but Cullen doubts this since it contains more oil, and also a sufficient quantity was seldom available. In some cases the use of whey rather than whole milk may be better.

Although some physicians had proposed milk as a remedy for all febrile states, Cullen considered it 'an ambiguous remedy'. Although useful in 'obviating and correcting a phlogistic diathesis . . . I have observed it to prove disagreeable to the stomach and often to excite the thirst it was intended to remove'. Cullen's practice was never to prescribe 'entire' milk in any case of fever. 'Entire' could mean either a diet restricted to milk only or whole milk. The consultation letters tell how frequently he recommended whey for his patients. Both uses of the word 'entire' probably apply.

Finally, he discusses the value of a milk diet in gout, both in prevention for those susceptible to it and in curing those already affected. It is emphasised that to be effective the replacement of all other animal food by milk should be continued for a long period and 'I am persuaded, that after an abstemious course for some time, it can hardly ever be safe to return to a free and full diet.

On animal foods

This section gives an account of 'food consisting of the whole, or of part, of the substance of animals'.

> The solid and fluid parts of the mammalia are so nearly of the same nature with one another, that the fitness of all of them for nourishing any of the other who live on animal food, and therefore the fitness more or less of all of them for nourishing the human species, can hardly be doubted of, and is very well established by much experience . . . We have only to examine the greater or less fitness of the several orders, genera, and species, for that purpose . . . That quality of animal substances fitting them to be aliments which first deserves to be mentioned, seems to me the degree of solubility in the human stomach (p. 356).

The solvent power of gastric juice varies in different animals and also in individual humans in whom 'it is manifestly different according to certain conditions in the aliments taken in. The condition especially giving more or less of solubility, is the different firmness of texture which appears in animal substances'. The species, sex, age, previous diet and exercise of animals affects the density or tenderness of the meat that they provide, and also the interval after death before the flesh is eaten. These factors are all discussed, as is later in the treatise the effects of different methods of cooking.

General considerations of aliments of animal origin are next discussed.

The first effect to be taken notice of is their giving, in the same proportion taken in, more nourishment than any vegetable aliments do. The latter can afford, as we have said, the whole juices of animal body, but certainly not in proportion to the quantity of them taken in; while animal substances that can be entirely dissolved in the gastric juice seem . . . to be entirely convertible as the expression is *in succum et sanguinem* [into juice and blood]. If at the same time they are in the smallest quantity less perspired they must greatly increase the plethoric state of the blood vessels [Cullen followed Sanctorius' views that animal aliments were in part lost from the body through invisible perspiration]. Animal food, therefore, is always ready to induce this state; and in growing bodies, such food will always favour, and probably hasten the growth: and although in adults, exercise and other means, by suppressing the excretions, may present it having this effect, yet it will always have a tendency to produce a plethora *ad volumen*. Moreover, as animal aliments for the most part introduce a greater proportion of oily matter, they are ready to occasion a larger secretion of oil into the adipose membrane, and thereby produce obesity (p. 365).

Then follows a consideration of the effects of animal foods immediately after ingestion.

Every kind of food taken into the stomach, as soon as it sets this organ to work, increases the action of the heart, and occasions a frequency of pulse; and if we mistake not, by the energy of the brain's being thus directed to the heart and stomach, a torpor in the animal functions, both of sense and motion, is induced, and often to a degree of sleepiness. . . These effects of food are more considerable from animal than from vegetable food. It seems also equally manifest that the feverish state during digestion is in proportion to the alkalescency of the animal food taken in, and that the degree of torpor induced, and the continuance of the feverish state, is more or less according to the quantity of food taken in (p. 367).

Now follows Cullen's most emphatic statement about diet.

. . . although animal food may be admissible by the human œconomy; and in certain circumstances of that it may be proper and even necessary; and therefore that, in many cases, it may be consistent with health: yet that, for the most part, a small proportion of it only is necessary; that the very temperate and sparing use of it is the surest means of preserving health and obtaining long life; whilst the large use of it tends to the production of diseases, and to the aggravation of those that from other causes may incidentally come on (p. 368).

Finally, the alimentary qualities of the flesh of many species of mammals, domestic and wild, of birds, of fishes and of other sea foods – lobsters, crabs, cockles and mussels – and of amphibia – frogs and tortoises – are described. Thirty-seven pages are given over to this subject of perennial interest to cooks, trying to provide tender and appetising meat for their families, and to innumerable individuals with digestive peculiarities, trying to find a food that suits them. Cullen provides a fascinating account of the folklore associated with eighteenth-century Scottish diets. He attempts to use the science of his day to explain the variations in the meats and also in the digestive capabilities of consumers. Nearly all of his explanations are nonsense and, indeed, only since the advent of molecular biology has it been possible to provide answers backed up by good science. But Cullen was right in presenting these problems to his students since doctors, then and now, are frequently asked about them by patients.

Alcoholic drinks

The account of the preparation and properties of these is curiously uneven and, for once, Cullen appears to have been influenced by the habits and prejudices of the urban professional classes. Whilst the account of foreign wines is as informative as that of most other aliments ales, the common beverage of most of the people, are treated cursorily; there is no account of home brewing, in sharp contrast to the account previously given of cheese-making. Whisky does not even get a mention, though it had been drunk in the Highlands for centuries and illicit distilling had become a well-known industry during Cullen's lifetime.

The effects of alcohol on people in everyday life and its uses in the management of patients are not discussed under aliments, but later in the *Treatise* in the section on sedatives. Here there is a concise account of the pharmacological properties of alcohol that could be read with profit by students today. This is now reproduced from vol. II pp. 315–18.

> Wine I have formerly considered as a drink, and have there said all that seemed necessary with respect to its preparation; and from the various causes of this we have endeavoured to explain its various conditions, particularly the different matters of which it may

consist; and, as depending upon these, the various sensible qualities that may appear in the different wines that are employed in our diet.

In all this . . . I have supposed, that what constitutes a wine is its containing a portion of alcohol; but the effects of this in diet I took little notice of, and mentioned only the effects that might arise from the other matters which might accompany it in the different wines appearing upon our tables.

It is, however, as containing alcohol that wines are to be considered as medicines; and the considering them as such we have reserved for this place, in which I have put them as narcotic sedatives.

That alcohol is such, can hardly be doubted; as, when only diluted with water so much that it can be swallowed, it shows the inebriating, intoxicating, and narcotic effects of other sedatives. When taken in small quantity, and much diluted, it does not indeed immediately show its sedative power; but, on the contrary, it may appear as a stimulant, cordial, and exhilarating liquor. As these operations, however, are in common to it with opium and other narcotics, they do not contradict our opinion of its proper sedative nature.

As in wine the alcohol is never in large proportion to the water at the same time present; and as in wine the alcohol is also blended with matters which diminish the force of it; wine can be, and is commonly, employed as a stimulant, cordial, and exhilarating liquor, more conveniently than alcohol could be in any other way. This explains why wine has been most commonly considered as a stimulant; but it is equally well known, that when taken to a certain quantity, it exerts all the sedative powers of alcohol or opium: and its medicinal qualities, according to the quantities in which it is employed, may be either stimulant or sedative.

Whenever, without fever, there is any languor or debility in the system, wine can be employed in moderate quantity with great advantage; as in most persons it is not only grateful to the palate, but also to the stomach: in which, if its acescent effects can be at the same time avoided, its cordial powers are immediately perceived, as from the stomach they are readily communicated to the whole of the system.

These are the virtues of wine employed in moderate quantities: And it is to be remarked by the way, that by its particular operation on the stomach it excites the action of this, and thereby promotes appetite and digestion: and passing further into the intestines, it does not so readily as other narcotics suspend the action of these and induce costiveness; but, on the contrary, by the mixture of its acescent parts with the bile, promotes the action of the intestines, and the evacuation by stool.

It may be further observed, that carried into the blood-vessels, by the alcohol it contains it promotes perspiration; and by the water and saline matters at the same time introduced, it certainly passes to the kidneys, and promotes the secretion of urine. Wine may produce all these effects, though taken in no large quantities; and they may be referred entirely to its stimulant powers of acescent qualities, which are in so far very commonly salutary.

It is difficult however to set the limits between its stimulant and sedative powers; and if the quantity of it be gradually increased, the latter gradually come on, and concurring with the former, produce at first a degree of delirium or inebriety, which is generally of the cheerful kind, and which occupying the mind, excludes all thoughts of care or anxiety: but the same sedative power carried on still further, renders the delirium more considerable, and gives the irregularity and confusion of thought which is the state of intoxication; and at length the sedative power entirely prevailing, the animal functions, both of sense and motion, are gradually weakened, and the person falls asleep.

In the first place, it will be obvious, that when the system is under any irritation increasing the action of the heart and arteries, the stimulant power of wine, even in most moderate degree, must be hurtful: and as there is hardly any irritation more considerable or more permanent than inflammation subsisting in any part of the body; so in all pyrexiae produced by inflammation, wine must be particularly pernicious.

We are also persuaded that all active haemorrhagies are attended with an inflammatory diathesis; and therefore it will equally appear that wine is improper in such cases.

But we proceed no further on this subject of the use of wine in diseases, as it may be governed upon the same principles we have laid down above with respect to opium; with this difference, however, that if the sedative powers of either are to be sought for, they are to be obtained more easily and certainly by opium than by wine; but where the stimulant powers of either are separately, or as combined with the sedative to be employed, the management may be more easy and accurate with wine than with opium.

Comment

A reader of Cullen's consultation letters and of his textbooks soon realises that he was a fine physician and a fine teacher and understands how his great reputation was established in his own days. Hopefully the short abstracts and brief summaries given above provide sufficient evidence of this for readers who have neither the time nor the opportunity to study his original writings. They should also show that Cullen held the study of alimentation to be of great importance for medical practice.

Cullen's patients and his students must have appreciated that his advice on dietetics was founded on years of observation of men, women and children, the food that they ate and their health. The advice was practical and sensible. Diets had to be related to individuals and one man's meat could be another man's poison. By far the greater part of his dietetic management of patients and of his recommendations for health is the same as that given by wise physicians today, two hundred years later.

Cullen gave his students a scientific background for his recommendations, based on theory. This was always presented with appropriate doubts. Phrases such as 'I am persuaded' and 'as far as I know' abound in his writings. His students were taken along with him on journeys of enquiry in which they were his companions. He is never the pompous professor dictating dogma. This is surely the reason for his great reputation as a teacher.

Unfortunately, the science of his day was inadequate and many of his attempted explanations are now known to be rubbish. Cullen and Black, his student and life-long friend, were both creative scientists in their Glasgow days. When each moved to Edinburgh, their creativity waned and had vanished by 1770. This may have been due to their energies being taken up by teaching and consultant practices, Cullen as a physician and Black's mainly in industrial chemistry. Without these pursuits it is possible that a new class of chemical substance (protein) might have been identified; Cullen was using appropriate words – caseous, coagulable, glutinous. Had they considered whether or not the therapeutic power of antiscorbutics was proportional to their acidity, they might have been led to the concept of a deficiency disease. Priestley's discovery of dephlogisted air, widely publicised in the early 1770s, might have led them to an understanding of the role of this gas in the inflammation (or, as we now say, combustion) of inorganic matter and in the animal economy, and so anticipated Lavoisier. It is worthwhile to consider sometimes the blindspots of scientists in bygone times; at least the exercise may lead to a realisation that we probably also have our blindspots which will appear strange to future generations.

It would be improper to end this paper on a carping note, dependent on hindsight. Cullen must have the last word, and here follows the conclusion of Part II of the *Treatise of the Materia Medica*, entitled *of Aliments*.

With respect to the most part of mankind, the different effects of aliment are not very remarkable; and though some excesses may take place, they are often transitory and unheeded: but it would be of consequence for men to know, that repetition may in time render these effects considerable and dangerous. It were well, that mankind was aware of the tendency which every kind of diet has to produce effects either immediately, or after repetition, unfavourable to health. It would, however, be difficult to give to the bulk of mankind the necessary instruction on this subject, and it would hardly be necessary to render it very universal, as it is not in many cases, and only in particular persons, that diseases arise from error in diet; but it is absolutely necessary that physicians who have the whole of mankind as objects of their attention, should study this matter; without which they cannot either perceive the causes of diseases, or direct the means of obviating them. In this business, however, I have often found physicians very deficient, from their great ignorance of the nature of aliments, and of the principles which should lead to the proper and necessary distinction of them. To supply this deficiency, and to give the necessary instruction, the foregoing treatise has been attempted; and though in some particular it may be both imperfect and mistaken, I flatter myself that it gives the necessary principles more fully and more justly than they had been given before, and at least points out the necessary particulars that must be entered into for ascertaining the nature of aliments more exactly. In all this I cannot have been too minute; and I cannot be of more service than by engaging physicians in a minute study of this subject (p. 432).

Soon after the author had begun to read his paper, William Cullen walked into the hall. He wore a large wig, a white cravat, white lace cuffs and an old College gown: he carried his well known cane. He agreed to answer questions about the dietetic advice that he gave to his patients and his dietetic teaching to students. This he did using the west of Scotland speech of his native Hamilton which contrasted with the author's Oxford English. The audience appreciated Cullen's visit and gave him a standing ovation. Not until he had left the hall did they realise that, in fact, they had been listening to Dr John Nimmo, the College Registrar, in disguise. The College has a tape-recording of the questions and answers.

8

Medical men, politicians and the medical schools at Glasgow and Edinburgh 1685–1803

ROGER L. EMERSON

Accounts of medical education in eighteenth-century Scotland all too often tend to start like this: Scotland in the seventeenth century was too poor and politically distraught to be able to create medical schools for which there was some clamour. By 1690 politics had put an end to Edinburgh's 1685 attempt to create a school and the economic and political problems of the pre- and post-union years prevented any further progress. The Principal of Edinburgh University from 1703, William Carstares, might plan a school on Dutch models but it was only later that the plans of an Edinburgh surgeon, John Munro, were successful. He wished for his son to be able to establish in Edinburgh a medical school on the Leiden pattern and what he wanted and worked for, Alexander Monro *primus* and the Edinburgh Town Council delivered between 1719 and 1726 'to save the liedges their money'.[1]

This story has now been somewhat modified. Stott has pointed out that Edinburgh was an important educational centre for surgeons by 1700.[2] Cunningham[3] and Guerrini[4] have commented on the medical teaching of Sir Robert Sibbald and Archibald Pitcairne, and Cunningham has noticed the rivalry between physicians and surgeons which seems to have marked medical progress in Edinburgh.[5] Lawrence has set out a three stage pattern of development in Scottish academic medicine and rooted this in 'an ideology of "cultural" improvement' which 'placed a particularly high value on practical knowledge and that esteemed natural science in this regard'.[6] Others have noted the generally progressive nature of Scottish education prior to 1700[7] and have commented on the scientism of that time.[8] Here I attempt to place the development of medical teaching in Edinburgh and Glasgow in a somewhat more realistic political setting than is usual.

From the 1680s until well into the 1800s Scottish politics were governed partly by ideological concerns which waxed, waned and changed but which had until the 1780s as a core a mixture of religion, patriotism, improvement and shame over Scottish backwardness.

Politics also involved an intense and usually organised effort to control, monopolise and even create jobs and places for the friends of those powerful enough to deserve consideration. Elsewhere I have described the ways in which patronage in Scotland was administered.[9] Here let me simply say that the family connections of the Campbells of Argyll, the Argathelians, and of the Patriot Party or the Squadrone dominated Scottish patronage politics until the 1760s. From c.1764 until c.1780 there were no leading or dominant figures in Scottish politics but in the universities the clerical Moderates, led by Principal William Robertson of Edinburgh University, managed to affect professorial recruitment in important ways. From 1778 and particularly after the death of Sir Laurence Dundas in 1781, Scottish politics were controlled ever more firmly by Henry Dundas whose regime lasted beyond his impeachment in 1806. Ideological conflicts might lead to rebellion but jobs were the stuff of life for most politicians. Monopolising them, parcelling them out, creating them and manipulating appointments were what kept the party managers busy.

Medical men in eighteenth-century Scotland were little different from other educated men who expected and sought places to which they felt entitled for a variety of reasons. Some expected to be favoured because of connections with leading political figures or because their families counted in local politics. Others found backers in Town Councils or medical and other corporations who needed to be placated. A few, like William Cullen, were so obviously meritorious that doing favours for them would buy the goodwill of many. The reasons for support might vary but throughout the eighteenth century, medical men clamoured for it and played politics as did lawyers, ministers, professors and those who received civil offices from the crown or municipalities. Physicians and surgeons agitated for the creation of new posts including university chairs. They plotted to obtain those which existed and were sometimes bitter losers. Medical education and the educators were immersed in politics.

One fact which politicised Scottish medical men was the small number of places available for them in Scotland. Few rural communities were able to support a physician, and among the physicians who practised in towns some were underemployed and hardly able to live as gentlemen on their professional earnings.[10] Surgeon-apothecaries were likely to be better off, but with about twenty-five apprentices booked in Edinburgh alone in any given year, those trained for the profession far exceeded those who could be employed in Scotland. More jobs became available after the first third of the century, but the increase did not keep pace with the growth in the number of competitors. Although practice also increased as cities expanded, emigration for many physicians and surgeons was a necessity. For the places which existed competition was intense and got fiercer as time went on. This was particularly true in the universities where the financial rewards soared with enrolments.[11]

A second fact of political life was the desire of every politician to monopolise control of as many institutions as he could manage. If the Duke of Argyll could pack Glasgow University with his men, he would have no embarrassing addresses to the Crown or Parliament, no undesirable University representatives in the General Assembly of the Kirk or the local synod and he would find more patronage at his disposal. He could then also embarrass the University's Chancellor, the Duke of Montrose, who was a political enemy. In an age without telephones, reliable men on the spot to look after one's interests were important. Their presence showed a patron's power and increased his prestige, which was no small matter. Accepting appointments entailed obligations which often held after a patron had lost power. To that can be traced much of the factious behaviour of Scottish professors during this time.

Eighteenth century Scots lived in a period of volatile politics. Allegiances could and sometimes did shift quickly among the members of the polite elite and then among their henchmen. Most men who sought and granted places were used to calculating their chances, as well as to hedging their bets. They kept an eye on the political scene and looked for chances or took them when they came.

But we should not think that politics was only about jobs. Ideological pressures were intense, especially in the periods 1660–1725, 1743–50 and 1790–1835. Politicians and their organisers (they had organisations by about 1715) were certainly interested in a man's political and religious beliefs. Throughout most of the period 1680–1780 they were concerned to appoint men in the universities who were in some sense improvers interested in making Scotland more modern, prosperous, polite and respectable. That meant that merit or perceived merits had to be weighed. Since politicians could not usually judge the skill and knowledge of medical men, they required the advice of others and, in the first instance, usually took that of physicians and surgeons who belonged to their connection. The Royal College of Physicians, the Edinburgh Incorporation of Surgeons and the Glasgow Faculty of Physicians and Surgeons, as well as prominent Scottish medical men in London often gave advice. Once the medical schools of Edinburgh and Glasgow had become recognized (c. 1740 for Edinburgh, c. 1760 for Glasgow), the Universities themselves and the city fathers had an increasing interest in ensuring appointments which would enhance their reputations. The benefits derived from growing numbers of students living and spending in the towns, and thus swelling the purses of those who catered for them, were always in view. Medical patronage, then, was no different from most other kinds of patronage which involved men of skill and learning. Many interests had to be considered including, of course, those of the legal patrons of the places which politicians wished to bestow. Patronage usually involved compromises and generally, at this level, arrangements were made by and for Scots without much interference from England.

There were a number of ways in which political influence bore upon medical patronage. Universities became more dependent on government grants. The obvious aspect of this was the growing number of regius chairs. In 1700, Scotland had about 63 professorships of which 8 were Crown appointments; whereas by 1800 there were 84, 24 of them being Crown appointments. Here financial dependence meant government control. The increasing number of men appointed through political influence politicised university senates and college corporations, and probably made government grants easier to come by. Edinburgh and Glasgow both got grants over the period. Glasgow also found subsidies in the tack of archibishop's teinds and indirect grants. At Edinburgh, funds went to salaries, the Botanic Garden and to buildings. In both places sinecure posts and offices which carried salaries were found for professors whose chairs were not in the gift of the Crown. All of this helped to secularise the colleges even though roughly the same proportion of laymen to clerics was maintained from 1690 to 1800.[12] In the working out of the relations between the municipal governments and the managers of the Crown's Scottish interests, city fathers were in general not entirely independent. At Aberdeen the evidence for this view is very good; in Edinburgh where less work has been done, this comment is more conjectural.

One way in which politics and politicians impinged upon the medical community and the universities can be seen in the creation of new places, among which were the fifteen medical chairs created between 1700 and 1793. There was always some value in aiding the universities. Politcans newly come to power, or consolidating their hold on things, created most of these new chairs, including those founded in the medical schools of Glasgow and Edinburgh.

By the 1680s the pressures on Scottish politicians to create chairs of law and medicine had grown as both lawyers and medical men had enhanced their status and organised stronger corporations.[13] By the 1680s there was also a need to placate professional groups and to buy political support for a monarchy in distress.[14] The first attempt to establish an Edinburgh medical school in 1685 reflected those conditions. Similar political needs had helped to create the Royal College of Physicians in 1681.[15] In both cases the Duke of York (later James II and VII) and his friends increased their support and put into the University three MDs (Sir Robert Sibbald, James Halket and Archibald Pitcairne) whose loyalty seemed sure. The Oath of Allegiance tendered to professors in 1679 had had a similar purpose, as did 'the Test for practising physicians' of 1684. The attempt to secure a new patent for the Surgeons' company in 1686 was perhaps also meant to insure the ascendency of Episcopalians loyal to James who would be willing to accept a Catholic prince as King. It was not only to preserve the rights of the surgeons.[16] The appointments of the three professors were probably not intended to be honorary since both Sibbald and Pitcairne were interested in teaching and either taught, or tried to do so, later in life. All these plans came to nothing in 1689–90. Of the medical teachers, only James Sutherland, the keeper of the College Garden and lecturer on botany, survived the purge of Jacobites and Episcopalians carried out in 1690 by a Visitation Commission. Sutherland not only survived but received further patronage in 1695, 1699 and 1710.[17] This came from governments which included men who had long known him and who in some instances shared his scientistic outlook and antiquarian interests.

The idea of reviving medical chairs was discussed by the Visitation Commissions which sat in the 1690s and is said to have been among the schemes which Principal Carstares long nourished. What we do know of the appointments made to Edinburgh chairs in Carstares' time suggests somewhat different interests at work; some were not seeking merely improvements by emulation of the Dutch.

The botany chair exemplifies the less than idealistic pressures which affected professorial recruitment. In 1705 Sutherland's chair went to Charles Preston, to whose brother George the government owed three years back-pay for being Surgeon-Major in Scotland. The Surgeon-Major continued to seek his dues. In 1712 George Preston succeeded to the chair of his recently deceased brother. In both cases the Prestons had the recommendation of the Incorporation of Surgeons and in both cases the Town Council chose the son of a Lothian laird who had been a Senator of the College of Justice. The Prestons were very well connected as well as being correspondents of London *virtuosi*. As late as 1714 George Preston was asking for military medical patronage to be 'enabled to improve the science of Botany'.[18]

In the chair of chemistry and medicine established in 1713 something similar can be found.[19] James Crawford, the Leiden MD who got the post, was friendly with Dr Pitcairne and with Squadrone politicians who in 1714 seem to have been willing to translate him to the new Glasgow chair of medicine.[20] He stood well with the Royal College of Physicians, which recommended him at Edinburgh, and apparently with Principal Carstares. Crawford may also have been related to professors at Glasgow who were Carstares' allies in the Kirk. No doubt he was a talented and well-trained doctor and chemist but his political connections also seem impeccable.

Politics involving the Edinburgh anatomy chair can be found in three contexts: the pre-history of the chair, the emulous rivalry of the Universities of Glasgow and Edinburgh and city politics in Edinburgh.

An interest in the university teaching of anatomy long antedated that expressed by John Munro in c. 1718 and the signs of politicking are clear. The Surgeons' company in 1705 appointed Robert Elliot to be its teacher of anatomy and gave him the use of its theatre. This was a move partly designed to protect a teaching monopoly. In the same year he was given a salary of £15 by the Town Council but was not appointed a professor, although he was made responsible for the 'rarities' in the University. In August 1708 he had conjoined with him Adam Drummond.[21] Drummond got appointments both by the Incorporation of Surgeons and the Town Council, as did John McGill who succeeded Elliot after the latter's death in 1715. Elliot received the title, professor of anatomy, within three years of taking office, but it was awarded to Drummond and McGill on appointment. In granting these titles the Town Council did not specify whether the professorships were to be held in the University or City of Edinburgh.[22]

That others had ideas about what could be done with an anatomy professorship is clear from letters to and from the Earl of Mar. Dr Archibald Pitcairne, physician to Mar's family, on 4 November 1708 jogged the Earl's memory about 'Adam Drummond his profession of Anatomie at Edinburgh . . . Wee stand in need of it extremelie, and he is most fit for it'.[23] Since Drummond already had an appointment from the Incorporation of Surgeons, this can only refer to a university post or to a professorship in the town and country such as had been held by Alexander Cunningham of Block in civil law and after 1716 would be enjoyed by Charles Alston, the King's Botanist. It was almost certainly a university chair which was at stake, and one from which Elliot would have been excluded since only Drummond is mentioned. Such a university post had already been sought in 'physick and anatomie' by the brother of George Erskine of Balgonie; that was probably what Pitcairne wanted for his protégé.[24] A creation of that sort would not have been welcomed by the Incorporation but it would have established the first medical chair in Edinburgh University since 1685. When in January 1709 Dr Pitcairne pleaded with Mar to send 'the patent without a salary', he almost certainly had in mind a regius chair within the College's walls.[25] Later Drummond did get a regius patent since in several places he is listed as a regius professor.[26] That designation is lacking in the case of his colleagues Robert Elliot and John McGill who replaced the former. McGill, the Deacon of the Incorporation, was elected professor of anatomy by the Town Council in 1716, and by his colleagues on 28 March 1717.[27] Behind these appointments it is not hard to guess at lines of influence. Elliot was Pitcairne's former student.[28]

Drummond was his friend and was related to other Drummonds who got patronage around this time. Among them was George Drummond who in 1707 had been made Accountant General of Excise, probably through the interest of the Duke of Queensberry who was then a member of the Scottish Privy Council.[29] Mar, as Secretary of State, may not have been able to get the requisite warrant for Adam Drummond. Perhaps the Chancellor, Lord Seafield, who supported another candidate, blocked him. In 1717 McGill may well have been paid off by the Argathelian interest. It had recently come to power in Edinburgh and elected the Provost in the years 1715–20 and 1723–4. One may well believe that John Monro helped to found the Edinburgh Medical School but one should recognise two things – the self serving character of his son's autobiography[30] and the background of activity to create a chair in 1708–9.

The second context in which the politics of the Edinburgh anatomy chair should be set is rivalry of Glasgow and Edinburgh throughout much of the century. What one got the other soon wanted. Edinburgh had been the first to teach botany but by 1704 Glasgow had caught up.[31] In the following year Edinburgh appointed Robert Elliot as its keeper of 'rarities' when he was elected public dissector of anatomy by the Incorporation of Surgeons. That gave him a place in its university. Glasgow, by the end of that year, had asked Mar to revive its medical chair.[32] Four years later, on 6 November 1712 the Glasgow professors resolved to petition Queen Anne for a chair of medicine.[33] By 22 December 1713 Edinburgh's Town Council had created a chair of medicine and chemistry for James Crawford.[34] Glasgow got its regius chair of medicine in 1713 and filled it in 1714 with Dr John Johnstoun after Edinburgh's professor, James Crawford, apparently decided not to take it.[35] It was also about 1714 that Glasgow began the regular teaching of anatomy. Early in 1720 when the lecturer was replaced by a professor of anatomy and botany who refused to teach anatomy, the Glasgow professors worried.[36] At this time it may well have been known that Alexander Monro *primus* would succeed Professor Drummond when Monro returned from his foreign studies.[37] That was what happened in 1720. By then Glasgow appeared to have sufficient resources to teach medicine but it lacked the students whom its Principal had expected to come into the city and it had teachers whose allegiance to the Principal and his political friends was greater than their interest in teaching. This criticism of Glasgow's teachers applied particularly to Dr Thomas Brisbane, a Leiden graduate, who was appointed by Squadrone men to the newly created regius chair of botany and anatomy.[38] The professor refused to teach anatomy – he hated the sight of blood and could not dissect without revulsion. That put paid to Glasgow's pretensions as a medical school until William Cullen moved to the city in the 1740s.[39]

In 1720 none of that would have been clear to men in Edinburgh. The appointment of Alexander Monro *primus* to the new University chair of anatomy in 1720 must be seen against a background in which men knew only that another Leiden doctor would assume the Glasgow chair of anatomy at about the same time. Brisbane's patent was dated 28 February 1720; Monro's, which could be more expeditiously issued, had come on 29 January 1720.[40]

Monro's appointment also had a third context. That is, the political one which brought to power within the city of Edinburgh Argathelian councillors and in the country the Duke of Argyll and his brother, Archibald Campbell, 1st Earl of Ilay. Argyll's party during the late 1710s and 1720s struggled with the Squadrone led by the Duke of Roxburghe.[41] By 1720 one of Argyll's supporters in Edinburgh was George Drummond who held city office continuously after 1718.

It has been suggested that Drummond, in cahoots with John Monro, changed the wording on Alexander Monro's appointment to establish formally that his chair was in the City and the University.[42] I would like to sketch an equally conjectural scenario which appears to me more probable.

By 1720 the Argathelians controlled Edinburgh Town Council, the body through which they tried to manage the University. By 1721 they had returned the MP for Edinburgh. In the general election of 1722 they won seats throughout Scotland but they had not clearly beaten the Squadrone until 1725 when Roxburghe was driven from office, or perhaps, until 1727 when George II and his ministers retained the Argathelians in power as Scottish managers.[43] As the political battles were won, Ilay and his brother gathered up what they could and consolidated power. In the process of doing so – and the process accelerated in 1725 when Ilay became Scottish Secretary in all but title – they interfered at all the universities whenever occasion offered. The St Andrews divinity chair had long scandalised the Kirk. Ilay tried to displace its occupant and to control appointments to the chairs of ecclesiastical history and Greek at St Salvator's. In Aberdeen his men took over the Rectorial Court at Marischal College in 1723 and he supported a College faction which opposed Principal Blackwell, a Squadrone supporter who was reluctantly forced into Ilay's camp by 1728. The Aberdeen Town Council had to agree to fill the Marischal College principalship and divinity chairs as Ilay wished and in a fashion they did not want. At King's College between 1717 and 1729 Ilay had only one opportunity to meddle with appointments. He seems to have failed to do so only because of insufficient time. Old Aberdeen, however, got a new burgh charter in 1725. Glasgow University was visited by his friends in 1726–7. Its Principal was disciplined and the College reformed. Ilay would have been eager to exert his influence in

Edinburgh.[44] His first chance to do so probably came in 1716 when William Wishart, long one of his supporters, became principal. His second came in 1720 when Alexander Monro *primus* was appointed.

If I am correct in seeing Glasgow and Edinburgh as emulous institutions, it would, indeed, have been a good thing for Ilay and his friends to have created a new chair in Edinburgh in 1720 and others in 1724 and 1726. This would have made life more difficult for Squadrone Glasgow. It would have gratified the Incorporation of Surgeons and those who wished to see better medical education provided in Edinburgh. Given the apparent interest in the establishment of a regius chair in anatomy eleven years earlier, this would have partially fulfilled that dream. Finally, creating an anatomy chair would fit with other things Ilay did at Edinburgh around 1726. These too should be considered.

In August 1724, just before the annual burgh elections held in September or October and before Provost Campbell left office, Edinburgh Town Council balanced the numbers of physicians and surgeons in the University by appointing William Porterfield to the new chair of the institutes and practice of medicine. The timing could hardly have been accidental. What Ilay wanted in an appointee can be seen in another such, brought in a year later. In 1725 Colin Maclaurin, who had supported Ilay's friends at Marischal College, was translated to Edinburgh's chair of mathematics. He had known Ilay since 1720. By 1726 he was giving advice to Ilay. In 1726 Maclaurin was in London arranging minor political matters for the Earl. He was the sort of man Ilay liked to place. In 1726–7 the Earl was also thinking about the principalships of both Edinburgh and Glasgow. He was clearly planning promotions and shuffles which would open a string of places so that as many as possible might be gratified. These schemes were made easier in 1727 when the King's death put at his disposal offices, such as chaplaincies,[45] held during the monarch's life. In 1729 he bestowed the Edinburgh Greek chair on what were surely political lines.[46] One should ask if and how the founding of the Edinburgh Medical School in 1726 fits into this picture.

The school had in a sense been founded in 1720 when Alexander Monro *primus* began to lecture on anatomy and Charles Alston started his extramural lectures on materia medica and botany. Although some instruction was provided in chemistry by James Crawford, the lack of input by a professor of medicine was a major deficiency. Although Porterfield could have undertaken this task he chose not to do so. From 11 October 1725 medicine was taught by two extra-mural lecturers at Surgeons' Hall, William Graeme and George Martine. Both sought posts in the University in 1726 and failed to get them. Martine was from St Andrews and was alleged to have had a Jacobite past. In the aftermath of the Atterbury Plot (1720–3) and the Malt Tax Riots (1725) such a man could hardly hope to get a place from Whigs like Ilay and Argyll. Graeme bore the surname of the Dukes of Montrose and may well have been even more politically obnoxious. We know that Graeme and Martine were oriented toward iatro-mechanism and anatomy, toward Boerhaave's medical system but not to chemistry.[47] And, we know that Graeme attributed their defeat to a 'party of men'. [48] Lord Ilay had very clear and definite interests in chemistry; in 1726 it was a set of four young chemists who became the University's first real professors of medicine.

For this to happen both Porterfield and Crawford had to vacate their chairs. Crawford had obtained the chair of Hebrew in 1719 despite the objections of George Drummond. He had not taught chemistry for some time.[49] He was probably also a client of the 1st Duke of Montrose, Chancellor of Glasgow University from 1714 to 1743.[50] In 1726–7 Ilay's friends were hectoring Glasgow's Professor Brisbane for neglecting his academic duties, and in 1730 they were still thinking of sacking him. Crawford's case was similar. So too was Porterfield's. Like Martine and probably Graeme, Porterfield was not from Edinburgh,[51] a fact which influenced Town Councillors who usually preferred their own men. Neither was doing anything of an improving nature which would recommend him to a political manager like Ilay. What we may ask did the Earl look for?[52]

Generally Lord Ilay looked for men who could help his political cause, but when left to himself he tended to pick those who shared his interests. He was a notable improver who looked after his own resources and those of his friends. He believed that doing so helped his country too. His improved estates had collections of exotic plants as well as newly planted hillsides and avenues. He could and did botanise with Linnaeus's system in hand. He was enough of a chemist to prepare his own medicines and seems to have dosed his friends as well as himself. He had at least two laboratories and some sort of chemistry set with which he travelled – a fact which makes plausible the account of his pre-1740 meeting with William Cullen.[53] A book collector, a *virtuoso* with a cabinet of instruments and scientific toys, Ilay was also enough of a mathematician to get a place in the standard directory of British mathematicians working in the Georgian period. A Leiden man who kept his natural philosophy up to date, he also claimed at the age of fifty-six to be reading excerpts from Latin and Greek authors daily. Ilay was an extraordinary (and today an underrated) man. It would have been surprising if the Edinburgh medical chairs had been created without his knowledge or intervention. There is no certainty that he meddled in this matter. But, the four young physicians who petitioned for the posts in competition with Graeme and Martine and who did get

the chairs were also chemists. Since November 1724 they had rented
the College Garden in which to grow their simples and were manufacturing pharmaceuticals in the College precincts.[54] All were Leiden
graduates. One, Andrew Plummer, was later to be defender of the
Earl's interest.[55] Another, John Rutherford, was known, albeit much
later, for his innovations in agriculture. Andrew St Clair, the third, was
a cousin of Lord Milton, Ilay's Edinburgh agent or *sous ministre*. They
would have seemed far more attractive candidates to Milton and to Ilay
or to those who wished to please them than Graeme and Martine.
Appointing them was likely to satisfy a number of interests. The town
would get a medical faculty endorsed by the political faction in power.
The Council was clearly interested in that although perhaps slightly
sceptical of the likely success of this venture.[56] Ilay in 1726 was able to
quash protests from other universities or corporations. The chairs went
to Fellows of the Royal College of Physicians and Graeme and Martine
were not Fellows. In the University, Fellows of the College of Physicians
would now outnumber members of the Incorporation of Surgeons four
to three, and their prominence would be underlined by the fact that the
new professor of midwifery held office in the town not the University.
But, the Surgeons had obtained one post and there was the near
certainty that in the future professors of botany, anatomy and midwifery
would be balanced by only three physicians in chairs of medicine and
chemistry. Finally the physicians and surgeons had equal representation
in the Senatus. It was an arrangement better explained by Ilay's
interests and way of operating than by the machinations of a retired
Edinburgh army surgeon with a dream about founding a medical school.

After 1726 the Edinburgh Medical School remained of interest to
politicians in the Argathelian party which in most years dominated city
politics until Ilay's death in 1761. Ilay was prepared to take advice on
appointments from medical men but he was also concerned to reward
the faithful. In 1756 the midwifery chair went as a political pay-off to
Thomas Young.[57] In the same year William Cullen came to Edinburgh
to teach chemistry and clinical medicine. This deal had been arranged
by Dr John Clerk, Lord Kames, Lord Provost Drummond, Ilay's
Edinburgh manager, Andrew Fletcher, Lord Milton, and other Argathelians. Ilay who in 1743 succeeded his brother as Duke of Argyll
'employed the weight of his whole interest in favour of Dr Cullen'.[58]
Behind those transactions were developments in Glasgow to which we
should now turn.

In 1720 Glasgow had not been far behind Edinburgh University in the
provision of medical education. After 1726 it was in the doldrums where
it remained until the mid-1740s. Favoured by Mar and the Squadrone,
the University of Glasgow was divided by political allegiances and by

religious leanings. These surfaced in 1727–8, in 1735, and in the fights over a new divinity professor in 1740 and 1743. Earlier the case of Professor Simson, who held the divinity chair from 1708 to 1740 and was twice tried for heresy, had also split the College.[59] In the background there was also a Squadrone magnate, the Duke of Montrose, as Chancellor waiting for the moment to revive his interests. That moment came, briefly, with the fall of Walpole in 1742. The return to power of the Squadrone allowed Robert Hamilton to secure the regius professorship of botany and anatomy.[60] To other chairs it brought Thomas Craigie[61] and William Leechman. The 1730s and late 1740s were not years in which the Crown's Argathelian managers had much inducement to favour Glasgow by creating medical posts. When one came in 1747 it was a lectureship in chemistry founded by the College itself for William Cullen. This was his first academic appointment and it presaged better things. Before discussing Cullen's accession to the chair of medicine we need to digress briefly to consider how different the recruitment practices were in Edinburgh and Glasgow.

The University of Glasgow was one of Scotland's three pre-reformation church foundations which had been revived as semi-autonomous institutions after the reformation while Edinburgh University was unique, being a civic institution founded and governed by the Town. Edinburgh Town Council had far less control of the affairs of its University than is often realised. The Crown's managers gave a great deal of advice about the choice of men for most posts, and made appointments to six chairs after 1768. The city's lawyers handed in leets or short lists for the chairs of humanity, history, Scots and civil law while the medical men expected to be consulted on the five non-regius chairs in the Medical School. Although the Senate had no statutory powers in the making of appointments the submission of its advice and that of the city's clergy was encouraged during Principal Robertson's term of office, and this advice often proved decisive. Of the twenty-nine chairs at the University in 1800 the Town Council effectively disposed of none without advice. In 1700 it was probably little more independent. The Council usually found its autonomy rooted in the factional divisions present in the political nation or in the nepotistic interests of its members. Edinburgh's Town Council certainly made appointments to suit itself but it was regularly guided by others in most of its choices. Cullen's appointment in 1755 was typical of most others throughout the century.

At Glasgow the Senate and College Meeting, afforced by the Rector and Dean, were the electing bodies. In 1800 in a faculty of eighteen, five were Crown appointees; no one was placed by private patrons and the city had no corporations able to affect recruitment except the clergy whose influence was sharply diminished after 1745. The Masters, if they wished, could ignore outside interference from the gentry and politicians. Politicians who wished to control Glasgow University had to build up within it a party interest. By the mid 1720s the Squadrone party had been doing that for a generation. In 1725 the Chancellor was the Duke of Montrose; the Rector was a Squadrone supporter as were the Dean and Minister of Glasgow, the Visitors of the College. Of the thirteen professors, all but two belonged to that party and at least three were related to the Principal. It is not surprising that Ilay in 1726–7 should have sought to cow this corporation. He gave it a new principal in 1727. Some professors were bought with small favours; two neutrals sided with him and a vacancy allowed him to bring in a man of his own, Francis Hutcheson. By 1730 Ilay could expect a majority in the College meetings but he did not have solid support until after 1746 when he returned to power after a four year absence. As we have seen, the Squadrone had added three men to the staff in those years and had helped the defeat of John Maclaurin's candidacy for the divinity chair in 1740 and 1743. William Cullen in 1744 came to a town and university in which party tensions were still high and the struggle for the control of Scottish patronage at London still unresolved. He also came to an institution in which deals could be made with the approval of the Masters.

James Moor, a protégé of the Earls of Erroll and Selkirk and the former tutor of Lord Kilmarnock, got the Greek chair in 1746. He bought it in a deal which provided an honorable retirement for its incumbent, Alexander Dunlop.[62] William Cross in the same year received the regius chair of law probably on the solicitation of Duncan Forbes of Culloden.[63] Cross's appointment had been opposed by his future colleagues who favoured Hercules Lindsay. Lindsay had sought it for some time and had boasted that Ilay would get it for him.[64] In 1750 he did. The moral philosophy chair in 1746 also went to Thomas Craigie a relative of the Squadrone Lord Advocate, Robert Craigie. These appointments are interesting because they show that in 1746 a number of people were dickering at Glasgow and that the masters were dealing with them rather independently. If Ilay were to recapture Glasgow's loyalty, it would need management and the placement of friends. Cullen was potentially if not already a friend.

William Cullen's initial 1746 deal with Dr Johnstoun, whose deputy he became, was typical of many such bargains. Cullen would teach for fees, the professor would keep the salary and perquisites.[65] The assumption in these cases was that deputies would have an inside track when the next appointment was made, even though there could be no promise about this as far as regius chairs were concerned. Cullen clearly impressed his colleagues who in 1747 made him a lecturer in chemistry and subsidised the building of his laboratory.[66] It was probably also clear to them that they were appointing a doctor who could teach medicine, botany and chemistry[67] – all subjects of interest to Argyll as well as to themselves. If the Duke had met Cullen by this time,[68] he may also have known of the doctor's interest in agriculture and of his belief that chemistry could and should be applied to industrial improvements. Those too may well have counted both in 1747 and 1751 when Cullen was made first a lecturer and then professor of medicine.

Argyll's chemical interests were not only medical and pharmaceutical. They also related to industrial problems as numerous letters throughout the 1740s show. In 1741 he was corresponding with Alexander Lind about the smelting of iron. Could peat be used to replace pitcoal and charcoal in this process? If it could, would the substitution be cost-effective and would peat prove to be less sulphurous than pitcoal? Lind's investigations into the composition, uses and properties of peat continued into the 1750s.[69] In 1742 Lind also was busy making 'comparisons of the weight of Lixeivial [sic] salt etc.', tests perhaps related to attempts to make porcelain and almost certainly to the search for native alkalis and bleaching agents. Argyll and Lord Milton were in some manner concerned with the Delf Potteries at Glasgow for which Lind reported working in 1749. A year later he wrote from London to Lord Milton saying that he, Argyll, the Earl of Hyndford and (Lord?) Falconer had visited 'a china manufacture at Bow and Chelsea'. He regretted that they had not been shown the materials used. Lind was later to work, as did Cullen, for the Board of Trustees.[70] In 1749 Argyll gave Lind the first of a number of legal posts which constituted his reward for doing improving chemistry. He was not alone in those activities. Others who pursued them were also in contact with Cullen by 1749 and probably by 1746. Glasgow university men would probably have seen Cullen's usefulness to them in the context of what Edinburgh improving societies were doing in the 1740s.

Until 1746 Edinburgh had two notable improvement societies – the Philosophical Society of Edinburgh (1737–83), a *virtuoso* group modelled on foreign societies and the Royal Society of London, and The Honourable the Improvers in the Knowledge of Agriculture in Scotland (1723–46), a society which was *sui generis*. In 1743 the Improvers authorised the publication of a volume of *Select Transactions*. These papers promoted agricultural experimentation, even calling for the establishment of a regius professor of agriculture in Scotland. Among the things which should concern such a teacher were 'the Principles of all Nature; *Earth, Water, Air* and the *Sun*'. The quote was from Varro but the reference was to the traditional four elements still recognised by laymen and chemists. Argyll and Milton had long been members of this Society and in 1743 would have been pleased to find in its *Transactions* fulsome praise for the Duke's work as an improver both of agriculture and industry.[71] Neither Milton nor Argyll is known to have belonged to the Philosophical Society but Milton had access to some of its papers – a privilege which its rules restricted to members.[72] During the 1740s the Society also dealt with matters of interest to Argyll. Some of Lind's work on peat was read to it; so too was work on lime and its uses (1742) and perhaps something on alkalis.[73] Those were only in part medical topics. The Society issued its offer to do free mineral assays for Scottish landowners in 1742. A year later it purchased a 'digester from Mr. Hauksbee' – another indicator of chemical interests and researches. In 1745 someone in Edinburgh even seems to have given a 'College of Chimie' whose outline Alexander Lind transcribed.[74] About the same-time the Society considered topics related to Scottish trade and to Glasgow in particular: a cross-Scotland canal, a map of the coasts of northern Scotland and the Northwest and Northeast passages which, if found, would give life to northern agriculture, industry and ports.

By 1750 at the latest Cullen was probably thinking about such issues. Certainly he was in touch with Philosophical Society members by 1749 when we find him writing to Lord Kames about both agricultural and chemical topics. He had already lectured on agriculture and its relation to chemistry. His connection with Arthur Martine (George's brother) also suggests that industrial chemistry had become of interest to him. Martine owned a brick and tile works in Fife and would have been concerned with the chemistry of glazes and alkaline substances.[75] Those activities formed part of the background to Cullen's two Glasgow appointments in 1747 and 1751. But, do they shed light on Cullen's relationship to Argyll and the latter's aid to him in 1751? I think they do but my case is circumstantial.

The Glasgow masters would have seen the usefulness of having such a man as Cullen within their walls. By 1747 they would have concluded that Argyll was back in power for the foreseeable future. Picking a man whom he would like would not hurt them. There are other reasons to think that these were not merely idle and general thoughts. The initiator of Cullen's first appointment was Alexander Dunlop whose family had supported Argathelian interests for a long time. In 1744 Dunlop had been the travelling tutor to Sir James Campbell who would have felt an obligation to take care of him and who had access to Argyll. In 1747 it was Dunlop's salary which was used to equip Cullen's laboratory. The deal was acceptable to the masters and to Principal Neil Campbell.[76] Beyond those considerations one can only guess at other connections in 1747. The case in 1751 is much clearer. By then men in Edinburgh who were Argathelians, Arthur Martine and the Duke himself, worked to secure for Cullen the professorship of medicine. That story has been well told by Arthur Donovan and we need only note that it was 'by the influence of [Argyll] with the crown [that] Dr Cullen was appointed to be the successor of Dr Johnstoune'.[77]

Throughout the 1750s and 1760s most of the Glasgow professors were recruited with much help from well-placed outsiders. That is apparent in many cases, but particularly so in the case of the successors to Cullen in the chair of medicine. By early 1755 it was clear that Cullen would seek translation to the Edinburgh chair of chemistry. To his Glasgow chair of medicine either Drs Thomas Hamilton or Joseph Black might be appointed and an additional vacancy would arise if Hamilton was promoted. In the mid-1750s Argyll's position in London was more than a little shaky because he was disliked by the Duke of Cumberland and the Duke of Newcastle who had succeeded his deceased brother, Henry Pelham, as head of the ministry in 1754.[78] Argyll's relatively weak position would have produced many applicants for these regius chairs. The atmosphere in which these vacancies were filled, or were assumed to be filled, is described by Tobias Smollett in a letter to Dr John Moore dated 11 December 1755:

> I am heartily sorry to find your Cause is so slenderly supported with the Duke of Argyle because, without his Concurrence or rather his creative Word, I believe no Professorship can be filled up. Merit is altogether out of the Question. Every thing here as well as in your Country is carried by Cabal; and in Scotland, the Cabal of the Campbells will always preponderate. The Time is fast approaching when all the Lands, all the Places of Honour, Power and Profit will be in the possession of that worthy Clan. Then you many exclaim *non Numinis sed Campbellorum omnia plena*.[79]

Smollett was wrong about merit. Robert Hamilton, clearly a good candidate, got the chair of medicine; Joseph Black succeeded him in the chair of anatomy and botany. Hamilton was not likely to have been favoured by Argyll had he been politically more secure because Hamilton's family had opposed the Argathelians on numerous occasions in the past. Argyll did prevent Hamilton's brother, Thomas, from filling the anatomy chair, ostensibly because he did not wish to have two family members in the corporation but more likely because he would not aid old enemies unless there was good reason to do so.[80] In 1757 when Robert died and Black became professor of medicine with Argyll's help, Thomas Hamilton got the chair of anatomy and botany.[81] This kept the Hamiltons' valuable collection of anatomical preparations in Glasgow. In 1781 that was a consideration which also facilitated the succession of William Hamilton, Thomas's son, to this chair.[82] Nine years later when William died, James Jeffray had to buy much of the collection in order to lecture credibly on anatomy. Each of these selections probably involved more politics than is now apparent. Why else would Cullen and Hamilton in 1756 have sent their resignations by express dispatch to Edinburgh? Even with Argyll's support, they and their replacements could not be sure that others might not find the means to get warrants issued before their own![83]

The Edinburgh Medical School during these years shows a similar pattern of political influence. The opinions of professors and political patrons were clearly of more importance than those of the city fathers. Robert Whytt got his chair in 1747 upon the resignation of Andrew St Clair. This initially may have been a deal worked out between Whytt and St Clair but Provost Drummond, with Argyll's consent, is said to have secured the post for Whytt. As in Glasgow, here too, a chemist was chosen.[84] Seven years later Alexander Monro *primus* arranged his son's succession to his chair with 'the Concurrence of all the Professors under whom [Alexander Monro *secundus*] had studied, and of all the students whom he had taught'.[85] What also counted was the Monros' collection of anatomical preparations. Cultural property of such value could not be lost, particularly when Monro *secundus* was a talented man. There seem to be no references to this transaction in Lord Milton's correspondence, but it is about the only Edinburgh medical appointment made between 1747 and Argyll's death in 1761 of which that can be said and, more particularly, it is the only one of any sort in the years between 1752 and 1757. Most of the medical appointments, like that of Thomas Young to the chair of midwifery in 1756, went to talented and well recommended men.[86] Not surprisingly, William Cullen's placement in 1755 was of a piece with the others. Again, Arthur Donovan's account of the transactions involved is one to which I can add little but emphasis.

Cullen was rewarded for work done and, in a sense, promised. The second interesting aspect of his translation and the negotiations which led to it is that the College men, perhaps for the first time, seem to have acted as a group to influence the choice of a professor and to set at least some of the terms on which he came. This points both to their importance to the burgh and to the prestige which the Medical School had gained in one generation.[87] The professors were to continue to make their views known and became the real electors to medical chairs from about 1763 to 1778 – that is from Argyll's death and Bute's retirement until Henry Dundas was able to monopolise political power in the city and eventually in Scotland. For nearly a generation the managers of Scottish patronage were willing and eager to accept advice from the intellectual community or were so weak and ineffective that they could not prevent that community from determining policy. Throughout that period and, indeed, until his death in 1790, William Cullen played a role in the choice of new professors at Edinburgh, Glasgow and even at St Andrews.

The first of the professors' appointments may have been that of Robert Whytt to the Edinburgh chair of the institutes of medicine in 1747; certainly the professors helped to determine the selection of men in 1766 when Cullen succeeded Whytt in the institutes of medicine and John Gregory followed Rutherford in the practice of medicine. William Hunter had approached Lord Bute on Cullen's behalf,[88] and also some of Cullen's colleagues and the medical students asked for his appointment. His move left a vacancy in the chair of chemistry. Since at least 1764 Cullen, Principal Robertson, other University men and some of the *literati* had been working to bring Joseph Black to Edinburgh. This they effected, again with the support of the students.[89] Two years later, in 1768, Dr John Hope, who had obtained the regius chair of botany in 1761 through the Earl of Bute, divided his duties and in effect sold his lecture course in materia medica. He offered it first to Dr David Skene of Aberdeen. When Skene refused to go south, Hope, his colleagues, including Cullen, and the Town Council passed the job to Francis Home who had long been seeking a place in the Medical School.[90] The next vacancy came in 1773. Then the Town Council asked the medical professors to give their opinions on the fitness of at least five men who sought to become the professor of the institutes of medicine. Cullen's influence on the ultimate choice of Alexander Monro Drummond, physician to the King of Naples, can be inferred from the anger and resentment long expressed by William Buchan, one of the contenders. Buchan deplored Cullen's views in print and is alleged to have thought of calling him out on the field of honour.[91] When the next appointment to the chair of the institutes of medicine was made, the Town Council through 'the Lord Provost [only] put a verbal question to the Medical Professors, asking whether they had any objection to Dr James Gregory?'. Gregory's father, John, had in 1766 been virtually chosen by John Rutherford to succeed himself in the practice of medicine chair. Rutherford in 1764 had refused to resign and make way for Cullen but had been prepared to do so for Francis Home who had then the interest of Lord Milton and Baron William Mure as had Cullen later. James Gregory in 1776 was acceptable to those with whom he and Andrew Duncan had taught as Drummond's deputy. Gregory was also supported by his father's old friends. The Town Council's proceedings in this case so angered Duncan that he raged in print saying that 'the magistrates should, as formerly, send to the professors a list of the candidates that might offer, requesting their opinions which of them they believed to be best qualified for discharging the duties of that important office in all its branches'. Failing that, they should have taken 'the opinion of the colleges of physicians and surgeons at large on the same question'.[92] Some of those who read his diatribe in the *Medical*

Commentaries may not have been surprised when Duncan a few years later sided with the Foxite Whigs. By then Principal Robertson, Cullen and others amongst the *literati* had drifted into the Tory camp of Henry Dundas.[93] In 1773, however, Duncan and Cullen had been close enough for the latter to recommend Duncan for the Chandos chair of medicine at St Andrews. 'I will pawn my credit upon it', wrote Cullen to Baron Mure, 'that he will make an ingenious Professor, and an able practitioner of physic' – as he did at Edinburgh after 1789. John Gregory expressed a similar opinion to the St Andrew's chancellor, the Earl of Kinoull.[94]

There is evidence pointing to Cullen's interventions in appointments at Glasgow in 1759, 1761 and 1764. He probably aided or tried to aid Adam Ferguson, Patrick Cumin and perhaps Thomas Reid, just as in 1751–2 he tried to arrange there an appointment for David Hume.[95] Black's successors in the chair of chemistry, John Robison (1766) and William Irvine (1768), were picked without apparent outside interference but they almost certainly had Black's endorsement and very likely Cullen's whose concerns with chemical theory they shared. In 1774 Black and Cullen were members of the committee which found Robison the fittest of those who sought the Edinburgh chair of natural philosophy.[96] Both Black and Cullen may have backed Alexander Stevenson who got the Glasgow medical chair in 1766. He was supported by the Royal College of Physicians and by his future colleagues.[97] The Crown would have found it difficult to appoint an undeserving man given the then flourishing state of Glasgow's Medical School. After (and perhaps by) that date Cullen no longer seems to have been of importance in Glasgow patronage, but his increasing reputation made him influential in other settings. Anyone who has gone through the Cullen manuscripts in Edinburgh and Glasgow cannot have failed to notice the number of letters which came to him from former students then in the army, navy, East India Company, hospitals and a miscellany of other British and colonial institutions. In many cases, behind those letters were others from Cullen recommending the appointments of these men.[98]

After 1776 the political scene in Scotland changed. Wilkes, the Americans and the anti-Catholic rioters of 1779–80 all made British elites more conservative in outlook. By about 1778 Henry Dundas's political machine had started to consolidate its hold over both Edinburgh and the country and he had begun to be indispensable to the ministry in London. He would remain so until his impeachment in 1806. By 1790 Dundas could and did use fears provoked by the revolutionaries in France to gain more and more control over Scottish institutions. During the reign of 'Harry the Ninth' the universities and medical schools were again politicized and professors and intellectuals lost the influence which came to them after Argyll's death in 1761. One marker in this process is provided by the Surgeons' attempts from 1773 to 1778 to establish in the Edinburgh Medical School a chair of practical surgery.

In 1773 John Rae who taught surgery and dentistry extra-murally asked the Incorporation of Surgeons to approach the Crown about the establishment of a 'Professorship of Surgery'. This he saw 'as necessary and useful towards perfecting the students of Medicine and Surgery in this Branch of their Education'. Nothing immediately came of this initiative to by-pass the University and the Town Council. Monro *secundus* convinced both his colleagues and the Town Council that such a chair would infringe upon his rights. Monro in 1777 made the Town Council join a chair of surgery to his chair of anatomy in an explicit fashion. The Incorporation's Deacon and Council did not think the chair they proposed would trench on Monro's rights so they petitioned the Crown through Sir Laurence Dundas, the city's MP. From 1776 until his death in 1781 Sir Laurence Dundas was engaged in a protracted struggle with his distant cousin Henry Dundas for the control of the burgh and for as many other electoral districts as either could secure. The Surgeons' scheme fell victim to this. On 21 May 1777 Henry Dundas assured them of his 'regard' but refused to aid them in establishing a chair of surgery. He could not support their request 'as they had applied to Sir Laurence Dundas and seemed only to ask his assistance in aid of Sir Laurences'. The petition came to nothing. When in 1778 the Incorporation applied for a charter to make it a Royal College, it did so through Henry Dundas. But thanks to the Monros no chair of clinical surgery could be created until 1803.[99]

The Edinburgh chair of surgery dates the beginning of Henry Dundas's meddling with the medical schools. Other appointments show that we should believe his 1801 boast 'that for twenty years past every professor at Edinburgh and St Andrews was "appointed either actually by myself or upon my recommendation"'.[100] At Edinburgh this means that he would at least have assented to the appointments of Alexander Hamilton (1780 midwifery), Daniel Rutherford (1786 botany), Andrew Duncan (1789 institutes of medicine), Thomas Hope (1795 chemistry), James Home (1798 materia medica) and Alexander Monro *tertius* (1798 anatomy). That is plausible in every case but that of Duncan.[101] There is no reason to doubt Dundas's claim since one can show his or his friends' constant intervention in university affairs. This was also true at Glasgow.

Glasgow at the end of the eighteenth century still had a Duke of Montrose (the third Duke) at its head. He was a loyal Dundas party member and an assertive one who could not distinguish the merely independent from the Jacobins. The last successful faculty recommen-

dation to the regius chairs of medicine probably came in 1780. It went to
William Hamilton who had been groomed for the anatomy post by his
father and who, like Alexander Monro *secundus* and *tertius*, inherited a
store of teaching aids. William Hunter in London had also solicited
support for him. Even so, the Duke of Montrose had a finger in the
pie.[102] Ten years later when the chair was again vacant, Montrose, for
political reasons, forced upon the University James Jaffray.[103] He was a
credible anatomist but not much of a botanist. In 1799 he virtually split
his duties, giving those in botany to Dr Thomas Brown. In 1789 the
medical chair went to T.C. Hope, Professor Stevenson's nephew, who
was made conjoint professor. Stevenson's family had been connected
with the Dundas family in politics since the 1740s.[104] This job would
doubtless have pleased the professors who in 1787 had given Hope their
lectureship in chemistry and materia medica. When Hope went to
Edinburgh in 1796, Robert Freer, a former army surgeon and Captain in
the Glasgow 'Armed Association', was preferred. The professors'
choice for the post, Robert Cleghorn, was excluded because of 'his
alleged attachment to Modern Politicks and his connection with that
Party here'.[105] That had not bothered the masters who in 1788 had
placed him in the lectureship of materia medica. In 1791 that post was
filled only after Montrose's allies in the College got assurances of loyalty
from Richard Millar, the appointee. Hamilton, Hope, Cleghorn and
John Towers, who came to teach midwifery in 1790, were rather better
men than Jaffray and Robert Freer, but the Duke of Montrose did not
think so. By 1801 Professor George Jardine could call Montrose 'an
absolute Dictator' with whom 'I have no kind of Connection'.[106]

There is much about the origins and early years of the Edinburgh and
Glasgow Medical Schools which remains unknown, obscure or conjectural. This paper suggests that we shift our conjectures away from
John Monro and Provost George Drummond to a wider political sphere
in which they were not principal players. If we do that, we may well find
that the Schools were as much the product of politicians working for
their own ends as of anyone else. They grew and flourished at least
partly because the third Duke of Argyll was an intellectual, a medical
and chemical amateur, an improver and a skilful manipulator of men.
So too were Lord Bute and the Moderates – those most effective in
securing places during the generation after the Duke's death. These
qualities became less marked after Dundas's rise to power in the late
1770s. To the character of individuals we must also add the emulous
striving of the Universities. Their efforts were also set against a
background of improving activities as well as a realistic politics of
jobbery. Neither could be played out exclusively in the burghs but
involved the nobility and gentry and a few, but very few, Englishmen.

William Cullen was very much at home in that world and could play politics with the best of them. We should remember his achievements as in part made possible by the politics he played in highly politicised institutions.

Acknowledgements

For permission to quote from manuscripts in their keeping I am grateful to the Librarians and Keepers of the Scottish Record Office, the National Library of Scotland, the Royal College of Physicians of Edinburgh, the Royal College of Surgeons of Edinburgh and the Universities of St Andrews, Glasgow, Aberdeen and Edinburgh and to the Marquis of Bute.

Notes and references

1. R.E. Wright-St Clair, *Doctors Monro: A Medical Saga* (London, 1964), 16, 28.
2. R.M. Stott, 'The Incorporation of Surgeons and Medical Education and Practice in Edinburgh 1696–1755', unpublished Ph.D. dissertation, Edinburgh University, 1984; 'Teaching from below: The Incorporation of Surgeon-Apothecaries of Edinburgh 1670–1707', paper to the Amer. Assoc. for the Hist. of Medicine, 1987, Dr Stott estimates that twenty to twenty-five apprentices were 'booked' in Edinburgh every year so that 75–125 were studying in the city in most years between 1695 and 1730; *ibid.*, 14.
3. A. Cunningham, 'Sir Robert Sibbald and Medical Education, Edinburgh, 1706', *Clio Medica*, 13 (1978) 135–161. The lectures which Cunningham describes were never given; see Sir Robert Sibbald to Sir Hans Sloane, 1706, Edinburgh University Library [EUL]. Letters from Sir Robert Sibbald to Sir Hans Sloane . . . transcripts from Sloane MSS in the [British Library]. Dc.8.35f49. Sibbald says there '. . . bot they [the students] were for the shortest way of some Modern Hypotheses, and would not allow the tyme required by me so I gave over the project. I printed then a Commentarie upon the Lex Hippocrates & his epistle to his son Thessalus, in which I show the Qualifications required in a good Physitian . . .'. The pamphlet is more polemical than Cunningham thought.
4. A. Guerrini, 'James Keill, George Cheyne, and Newtonian Physiology, 1690–1740', *Jnl. of the Hist. of Biology* 18 (1985), 247–66; 'The Tory Newtonians: Gregory, Pitcairne, and Their Circle', *Jnl. of Brit. Studies* 25 (1986), 288–311; 'Archibald Pitcairne and Newtonian Medicine', *Medical History* 31 (1989), 70–83; 'Scottish Medical Men and the English Medical Profession, 1680–1730', forthcoming.
5. A. Cunningham, typescript of an as yet unpublished paper which Dr Cunningham graciously allowed me to read. See also his 'The Medical Professions and the Pattern of Medical Care: The Case of Edinburgh, c. 1670–c. 1700' in *Heilberufe und Kranke im 17 und 18 Jahrhundert*, eds W. Eckart and J. Geyer-Kordesch (Munster, 1982), 9–28.
6. C. Lawrence, 'Ornate physicians and learned artisans: Edinburgh medical men, 1726–1776' in *William Hunter and the eighteenth-century medical world*, ed. W.F. Bynum and Roy Porter, (Cambridge, 1985), 153–176, 174.

7. E.G. Forbes, 'Philosophy and Science Teaching in the Seventeenth Century' in *Four Centuries: Edinburgh University Life 1583–1983*, ed. G. Donaldson (Edinburgh, 1983), 28–37; C.M. Shepherd, 'Newtonianism in Scottish Universities in the Seventeenth Century' in *the Origins and Nature of the Scottish Enlightenment*, eds. R.H. Campbell and A.S. Skinner (Edinburgh, John Donald, 1982), 65–85.

8. R.L. Emerson, 'Natural philosophy and the problem of the Scottish Enlightenment', *Studies on Voltaire and the eighteenth century* (1986), 242: 243–91; 'Science and Moral philosophy in the Scottish Enlightenment' in *Oxford Studies in the History of Philosophy*, vol. 1: *Studies in the Philosophy of the Scottish Enlightenment*, ed. M.A. Stewart (Oxford, 1990), 11–36; P. Wood, 'Science and the Aberdeen Enlightenment' in *Philosophy and Science in the Scottish Enlightenment*, ed. P. Jones (Edinburgh, 1988), 39–66; 'Science and the pursuit of virtue in the Aberdeen Enlightenment', Stewart, *ibid.*, 127–150.

9. R.L. Emerson, *Professors, Patronage and Politics: The Aberdeen Universities in the Eighteenth Century* (Aberdeen University Press, 1992).

10. R.M. Stott, 'The Medical Practice of George Chalmers, M.D.', *Archiveria* 10 (1980), 51–67; B. Seton, 'Aesculapius in Fife: a Study of the Early Eighteenth Century', *Scot. Hist. Rev.* 19 (1922), 180–9.

11. J.B. Morrell, 'The University of Edinburgh in the Late Eighteenth Century: Its Scientific Eminence and Academic Structure', *Isis* 62 (1971), 158–71. My own studies of the Scottish professoriate suggest that what Morrell found at Edinburgh was true elsewhere, particularly if total income figures are included. By the second half of the century most professors had incomes well over £150. See Emerson (n9).

12. About a third of the professors qualified initially or eventually became ministers of the Kirk. The number did not shrink during the century.

13. R.G. Cant, 'Origins of the Enlightenment in Scotland: the Universities' in Campbell and Skinner (n7), 42–64; Emerson (n8; 1986), 252–5.

14. H. Ouston, 'York in Edinburgh: James VII and the Patronage of Learning in Scotland, 1679–1688' in *New Perspectives on the Politics and Culture of Early Modern Scotland*, eds. J. Dwyer, R.A. Mason, A. Murdoch (Edinburgh, n.d. [1982]), 133–35.

15. W.S. Craig, *History of the Royal College of Physicians of Edinburgh*, (Oxford, Blackwell, 1976), 39–69.

16. Ouston (n14) discusses all these developments.

17. H.R. Fletcher and W.H. Brown, *The Royal Botanic Garden Edinburgh, 1670–1970* (Edinburgh, 1970), 11–18.

18. Minute Books of the Royal College of Surgeons, vol. 3, 8 November 1705; 3 August 1712; Fletcher and Brown (n17), 26–36. George Preston to the Earl of Mar, 24 April 1707, Historical Manuscripts Commission [HMC], *The Manuscripts of the Earl of Mar and Kellie* (London, HMSO, 1904), 1:388. Preston's brother was a respected botanist and friend to Sir Robert Sibbald but his appointment would have helped a family to whom the government was indebted. George Preston to Mar, 18 November 1707: Col. George Preston to Mar, 12 December 1707, Mar and Kellie Manuscripts, Scottish Record Office [SRO], GD124/713; 730; GD124/15/1122.

19. W.P. Doyle, 'James Crawford M.D. (1682–1731)', pamphlet in *Scottish Men of Science* series (Edinburgh, History of Medicine and Science Unit, 1981).

20. Principal William Carstares to Principal John Stirling, 21 January 1714, Glasgow University Library [GUL], Murray MS 650/I. Carstares reported that the Edinburgh professors had told Crawford that he could accept the Glasgow chair if he wished. The Earl of Mar recommended Dr John Johnstoun on 6 March 1713; *ibid.* In 1715 Edinburgh University asked Montrose 'that the office of the first of

H.M. physicians in Scotland shall be annexed to the said professorship [of medicine and chemistry]'. EUL Laing MS II, 676.

21. Adam Drummond is incorrectly identified by Alexander Bower as the brother of George Drummond, Edinburgh's famous eighteenth-century Lord Provost: *The History of the University of Edinburgh*, 3 vols, (Edinburgh, 1817–30), 1: 185.

22. J. Struthers, Historical Sketch of the Edinburgh Anatomical School (Edinburgh, 1867), 12–17; E.A. Underwood, *Boerhaave's Men at Leyden and After* (Edinburgh, 1977), 94, 103–5.

23. Archibald Pitcairne to the Earl of Mar, 4 November 1708, *The best of our owne: Letters of Archibald Pitcairne, 1652–1713*, ed. W.T. Johnston (Edinburgh, 1979), 54–5.

24. 'Pray tel George Erskine of Balgownies brother, to whom I should have wrote e're now had I had time, that what he proposes for himself as to a profession of physick & anatomie is now impracticable, but I shall be very glade if I can serve him in anything else, tho I see nothing that offers at present.' Mar to James Erskine, Lord Grange, 5 February 1708; SRO MS GD124/15/754/6.

25. 'I must once again presume to recommend Adam Drommond to Your Lordship I hear My Lord Seafield is setting up for one Abercrombie, who, I know, is vastlie unfit for the profession of Anatomie. Rather than the affaire be spoilt, be pleas'd to send the patent without a salary.' Pitcairne to Mar, 24 January 1709, Johnston (n23), 56.

26. There is no notice of any of the University medical teachers in the various editions of John Chamberlayne's *Magnae Britanniae Notitia or the Present State of Great Britain* until 1724 when 'Mr. Adam Drummond' is listed as '*Regius* Professor of Anatomy'. In 1725 'Mr. Adam Drummond Surgeon and Prof. R of Anatomy' appears in the list of those who in 1724 'contributed to Augmenting of the Physiological Library'. If this was a newly conferred title it may have come as compensation when Drummond resigned in favour of Alexander Monro. It may also mean that at some other time between 1709 and 1719 plans to promote the teaching of anatomy within the University had been made and failed to come to anything. The 1727 list gives James Crawford as 'Professor of Medicine, and of the Oriental Languages' and notes the presence of Professors St Clair and Plummer but not of Rutherford and Innes. Drummond and Monro, but not George Preston, are listed but the town's new professor of midwifery, Joseph Gibson, is not noticed. Not until 1750 did this work print an accurate list of the medical school professors. I thank Dr Michael Barfoot for some of this information. See also: *Magna Britanniae Notitia* (London, 1724), Part II, Book III, 12; EUL, DE 10, 127.

27. Struthers, (n22) 12–15.

28. See n22.

29. There is no reliable or full account of George Drummond but see M. Hook *et. al. Lord Provost George Drummond 1687–1766* (Edinburgh, Scotland's Cultural History Unit, 1987).

30. This is documented in R.L. Emerson, 'The Philosophical Society of Edinburgh, 1737–1747', *Brit. Jnl. for the Hist. of Science*, 12 (1979), 154–91, 157, 161–171. The autobiography, boastful as it is, also shows us a young man well connected to London surgeons, chemists and other scientists and with friends in Leiden and Paris; Alexander Monro, primus, ed. H.D. Erlam, *Univ. of Edin. Jnl.* 17 (1953–5), 77–105, 81–2.

31. A.D. Boney, *The Lost Gardens of Glasgow University* (London, Christopher Helm, 1988, 31–4. A 'physick garden' had been projected in Glasgow since 1701; *Early Letters of Robert Wodrow 1698–1709*, ed. L.W. Sharp (Edinburgh, 1937, Scot. Hist. Soc., 3rd series, 24), 184 n1.

32. Principal John Stirling to the Earl of Mar, 3 December 1705, in HMC
    (n18), 240. In this letter Stirling said that if 'medicine were revived
    there would be no lack of students, even from England and elsewhere'.
33. J. Coutts, *A History of the University of Glasgow* (Glasgow, 1909),
    484.
34. A. Grant, *The Story of the University of Edinburgh*, 2 vols (London,
    1884), 1:296–8; Grant noted that Cambridge also got a chemistry chair
    in 1713.
35. See n20.
36. J.D. Mackie, *The University of Glasgow 1451–1951* (Glasgow, 1954),
    169–70.
37. Underwood (n23), 103.
38. J.B. Neilson (ed.) *Fortuna Domus* (Glasgow, 1952), 297; Mackie
    (n36), 170; Rector Mungo Graham of Gorthy to Principal John
    Stirling, 3 and 7 February 1719, Murray MS 651 (n20).
39. Students petitioned for the anatomist to teach and the faculty members
    demanded it in 1721. In 1727 and 1729 efforts were made to get
    anatomy taught, efforts which succeeded in 1730. Robert Dundas to
    Principal Stirling, 28 November 1721, Murray MS 650 (n20); Coutts
    (n33), 485–6; Robert Wodrow, *Analecta or Materials for a History of
    Remarkable Providences . . .* 4 vols (Edinburgh, Wodrow Society,
    1842), 4:28; H.M. Public Record Office SP 54/17/68. In the latter
    Ilay, who had been trying also to extrude Johnstoun, wrote to someone
    unknown 'I met with two things very diverting at Glasgow, one was
    that one Dr. Johnson had been under a prosecution before the late
    Commission [of the General Assembly of the Kirk] for having said
    that the Moon was an irregular bitch, which the other party said was
    speaking irreverently of that glorious luminary. The other matter was,
    that there is a Professor of Anatomy [Brisbane] there put in by our late
    Scotch administration who has a very extraordinary defect for one of
    his trade, viz. that he cannot bear the sight of blood nor of a dead
    corpse'. I thank Dr Andrew Cunningham for this reference.
40. Brisbane's Commission of Appointment is printed in Boney (n31),
    289–90.
41. R. Sedgwick *The History of Parliament: The House of Commons 1715–
    1754*, 2 vols (New York, Oxford University Press, 1970), 1:389–9; *The
    Lord Provosts of Edinburgh 1296 to 1932*, ed. T.B. Whitson (Edin-
    burgh, 1932), 60–5.
42. Underwood (n22), 105.
43. Segwick (n41), 1:34.
44. The cases listed are discussed in Emerson (n9).
45. *Ibid*.
46. Ilay refused to bestow this place on the son of the Rev. William Alston
    but gave it instead to William Scott, junior, son of the first man to hold
    the chair. Andrew Fletcher, Lord Milton, to Ilay, n.d. [1729], National
    Library of Scotland [NLS], Saltoun Correspondence SC 47 ff 176–9.
47. Martine's father was deprived of office after 1690; George is said to
    have rung the St Andrew's bells for the Pretender in 1715. See 'George
    Martine' in *The Dictionary of National Biography*. Martine's brother
    Arthur was later to claim that George's teaching at Surgeons' Hall had
    succeeded 'against a greater opposition' than William Cullen was likely
    to encounter from his professional colleagues in the winter of 1755–6.
    William Wilson to Cullen, 20 September 1755, Glasgow University
    Library [GUL], Thomson Cullen Papers 2255/73. That suggests that
    Martine and Graeme had been opposed by the University men while
    they taught – a not unlikely case since Martine was something of a
    chemist and anatomist and, thus, likely to poach on both Crawford's
    and Monro's territory. Martine in letters to James Douglas, 11 June

1733 and 4 August 1735 mentions lectures on the heart delivered in Edinburgh in 1725. GUL MS Gen.505(12), D626/1; D626/3; [W. Graeme] *An Essay for Reforming the Modern Way of Practising Medicine in Edinburgh* (Edinburgh, 1727), 25–7, gives a brief account of their course on 'the whole Art of Medicine' taught 'in *English* as well as in *Latin*'. In this course 'Surgery is fully explain'd', pp. 25–7.

48. Graeme, 1727 (n47), 4.
49. Doyle (n19), 4.
50. Unless he had stood well with Montrose and his friends, there would have been no point in contemplating a move to Glasgow in 1714 or in asking for a sinecure office in 1715. Such ties would account for Drummond's opposition.
51. He was from an Ayrshire or Renfrewshire family – Porterfield of Halfland or Haplands.
52. The following paragraph is based on my forthcoming paper, 'The Scottish Scientific and Medical Patronage of Archibald Campbell, 3rd Duke of Argyll 1723–1761'.
53. J. Anderson, 'Cursory Hints and Anecdotes of the late Doctor William Cullen of Edinburgh' in *The Bee or Literary Intelligencer* (1790–1): 1: 1–14, 45–56, 121–5, 161–6.
54. Minutes of the Professor of Medicine and Partners of the Chemical Elaboratory in Edinburgh, EUL, Gen 1959. The minutes run from 25 January 1731 to 1734; see also R.G.W. Anderson, *The Playfair Collection and the Teaching of Chemistry at the University of Edinburgh 1713–1858* (Edinburgh, 1978), 8, 15 n40.
55. In 1742 Plummer's refusal to vote for the Squadrone directors of the Bank of Scotland was reported to Tweeddale. Thomas Hay to the Marquis of Tweeddale, 27 April 1742, NLS, Yester Papers 7046 f100.
56. Writing to William Cullen on 3 February 1756, George Drummond said of these appointments, 'we were only making a tryal, and were somewhat uncertain about its success and Yet, they thought themselves favoured by The town Council in giving them a preference in our choice, to another sett who petitioned Us to appoint them'. GUL, Thomson Cullen MS 2255.
57. Professor John Anderson to Baron William Mure of Caldwell, 8 January 1763, printed in *Selections from the Family Papers Preserved at Caldwell* [ed. William Mure of Caldwell] 2 vols in 3, Maitland Club, Glasgow, 1884, vol. 1, part II: 163–4. Anderson was seeking to have a regius chair in midwifery created for John Moore. 'Similar to what was lately done for Dr Young in Edin^r.' He did not ask for a large stipend since the possession of the place would be 'much greater than five times the sum [salary] given annually' since it would bring in class fees, perquisites, improved practice and 'entitle his wife to 25£ a year & c. from the Widows' Fund'.
58. R. Chambers, *A Biographical Dictionary of Eminent Scotmen* 4 vols (Glasgow, 1856), 2:28.
59. In 1727–8 the Squadrone party Masters had tried to prevent the appointment of Neil Campbell to the Principal's chair: Lord Milton to Ilay, 1 December 1727, EUL, Saltoun MS SC 35. In 1735 George Ross, a relative of Lord Ross, an Argathelian, was chosen to succeed his father, Andrew, in the Latin chair. The 1740 and 1743 contests for the divinity chair pitted religious liberals who backed the successive candidacies of Michael Potter and William Leechman against John Maclaurin. For Potter were: *Montrose*, the Chancellor; *Graham* of Dougalston, Rector; Robert Simson, Francis Hutcheson, John Loudon, *Charles Morthland, William Anderson, Thomas Brisbane*. Against him were: William Forbes, *John Johnstoun*, Principal Neil Campbell, George Ross and *Robert Dick*. For Leechman were: *Rector*

George Bogle, Alexander Dunlop, *Charles Morthland*, Robert Simson, Francis Hutcheson, George Ross, *Robert Hamilton*. Against him and for Mclaurin were: Principal Neil Campbell, John Loudoun, William Forbes, *John Johnstoun, Robert Dick, William Anderson*. Colin Maclaurin appealed to Squadrone politicians to support his brother in 1743. Names of the Squadrone men have been italicised. These contests split the political factions, but outside the College Ilay supported Maclaurin in 1740 but not, perhaps, in 1743. The Squadrone in 1740 backed Potter and Leechman in 1743. Coutts (n33), 236–7; Glasgow faculty minutes, Glasgow University archives [GUA] 11 February, 20 March, 4 April, 17 June 1740; 29 November 1743–12 January 1744; Neil Campbell to Lord Milton, 1740; Archibald Campbell to Lord Milton, ?December, 1743; NLS, Saltoun Correspondence, SC 82 f51–2; SC 96f; Colin Maclaurin to Andrew Mitchell, 22 November, and 17 December, 1743 reprinted in *The Collected Letters of Colin MacLaurin*, ed. S. Mills (Nantwich, Shiva Publishing Co., 1982), 114–8; Thomas Hay to Marquis of Tweeddale, 26 November 1743, NLS, Yester Papers (n55), 7059/63. The Simson Case still awaits its historian but see *State of the Processes Depending against Mr. John Simson . . .*, ed. John Dundas (Edinburgh, 1728); J. Cunningham, *The Church History of Scotland*, 2 vols (Edinburgh, 1859), 2:405–14. Ilay and his friends worked to keep Simson in his University chairs, Charles Erskine to My Lord [?Ilay], 8 May 1729, NLS, Erskine-Murray MSS, 5073/128.

60. Thomas Hay to Tweeddale, 13 April 1742; Robert Dundas to Tweeddale, 15 April 1742; William Anderson to Tweeddale, 11 June 1742, NLS, Yester Papers 7046 ff39; 61; 704 f127.

61. Thomas Craigie had tried to secure the Edinburgh University mathematics chair in 1746 with the support of Lord Cathcart; this place he got through the efforts of Robert Craigie, the Squadrone Lord Advocate. He had since 1741 held the regius chair of Hebrew at St Andrew's which probably came to him through David Scot of Scotstarvit, after 1738 an opposition Whig allied to the 2nd Duke of Argyll but not to Lord Ilay.

62. Moor's principal patron, Selkirk, was a friend of Ilay; Dunlop had long been one of Ilay's allies in the College; John Stuart Shaw, *The Management of Scottish Society 1707–1764* (Edinburgh, 1983), 98.

63. Duncan Forbes to the Marquis of Tweeddale, 13 November 1745, NLS Yester Papers, 7070/22.

64. William Anderson to the Marquis of Tweeddale, 26 September 1744, NLS, Yester Papers, 7063/135–6.

65. A. Donovan, *Philosophical Chemistry in the Scottish Enlightenment* (Edinburgh, 1975), 49–50; Cullen's former dependence on the Hamilton interest in 1746 would have made him a political neutral and one easily able to cooperate with Professor Hamilton in his teaching.

66. GUA, Glasgow Faculty Minutes, 5 and 28 January, 11 February, 1 April 1747.

67. This account ignores his associate, John Carrick (d.1750), who was related to Professor John Simson and who also aided Robert Hamilton.

68. See n53 and D. Guthrie, 'William Cullen, M.D. and His Times' in *An Eighteenth Century Lectureship in Chemistry*, ed. A. Kent (Glasgow, 1950), 50.

69. Emerson, (n30), 187 n103, 188 n113; See also *The Scots Magazine*, September 1749, 487; John Thomson, *An Account of the Life, Letters, and Writings of William Cullen, M.D.*, 2 vols, (Edinburgh, 1859), 1:598.

70. Ibid, Emerson.

71. The Improvers' interests in experiments and its scientism are discussed in R.L. Emerson, 'Science, Society and Morals in Scotland 1700–1740', forthcoming.

72. '. . . Account of the Materials of which it is made, the way of burning or calcining Limestone . . . by Mr. [Alexander] Lind'; 'Of the nature & Vertues of Peats'; 'An Experiment upon the Motion of the Sap in Trees', NLS, Saltoun Papers, Miscellaneous MSS, SMisc 59b; SMisc. 54. Other papers in this last set probably belong to the Philosophical Society including 'Memorandum about Iron', etc.

73. References to the Society can be found in: Emerson (n30) and in R.L. Emerson, 'The Philosophical Society of Edinburgh, 1748–1768', *Brit. Jnl. for the Hist. of Sciences* 14 (1981), 156. Cullen joined the Society c.1749–56 becoming a vice-president in 1767.

74. NLS, Saltoun Misc. 54.

75. I thank Mr Robert Smart, Keeper of Manuscripts, St Andrews University, for this information.

76. Dunlop's 1744 appointment to the chair of oriental lanaugages was contested by the Squadrone politicians. 'Copy of Letter from University to Mr. Robt Craigie, King's Advocate', GUA 47463; J. Rendall, *The Origins of the Scottish Enlightenment* (London and New York, 1978), 57–8; Andrew Mitchell to Marquis of Tweeddale, 4 October 1744, NLS, Yester Papers 7064 f12–3. Donovan (n65), 63.

77. Donovan (n65), 50–69; Chambers (n58), 2:26; Coutts (n33), 487.

78. Shaw (n62), 180.

79. Tobias Smollett to John Moore, 11 December 1755 in *The Letters of Tobias Smollett*, ed. L.M. Knapp (Oxford, Clarendon Press, 1970), 42. ('All things are full not of divine power but of Campbells'.)

80. William Ruat to Robert Simson, 4 January 1756, GUA 30485.

81. Scroll, Lord Milton to the Duke of Argyll, 9 December 1756, NLS, SC 16694 f114.

82. Coutts (n33), 499–500.

83. Cullen obtained his conjoint appointment with Plummer at Edinburgh in November 1755 but he did not immediately resign his Glasgow chair. This angered Argyll who had told Newcastle that both Cullen's and Hamilton's chairs were vacant and that warrants were to be issued for patents to Thomas Hamilton and Joseph Black. These were drawn in February or March 1756 and the patents were issued and sent to Scotland by December 1756. Cullen's motive was less likely to have been private pecuniary gain than a desire to be absolutely sure that Black and Hamilton would be chosen. That uncertainty was rooted in the political processes by which regius chairs were filled. William Ruat to ? [Robert Simson] 11 March 1756, GUA 30492; Lord Milton to the Duke of Argyll, 9 December 1756, NLS SC 16694II f89.

84. Professor Andrew St Clair died on 25 October 1760 not earlier as is often said. Whytt is said to have come to the chair of the institutes of medicine through the efforts of his colleagues and George Drummond. His political credentials and ties were also good. In 1743 he married Louisa Balfour, the sister of John Balfour printer to the University. Another brother-in-law, James Balfour of Pilrig was made Sheriff-Substitute of Edinburgh in 1748. A. Dalzel, *History of the University of Edinburgh*, 2 vols (Edinburgh, 1862), 2:418; R.K. French, *Robert Whytt, The Soul, and Medicine* (London, 1969), 8. If Argyll did have a hand in this, he picked a man whose writing in the 1740s had been largely chemical as they continued to be well into the 1750s.

85. Wright-St Clair (n1), 69–72.

86. See n57.

87. Wright-St Clair (n1, 70) says that Monro *primus* in 1754 estimated that medical students alone brought into the city 'at least £10,000' a year.

88. Cullen's move to the chair of the institutes of medicine was a complicated business designed to bring Black to Edinburgh and to replace Professor Rutherford who wanted to see his chair go to Francis Home or, later, to John Gregory. The schemes played out over a four year period 1764–8. By then Black had come; Home and Gregory had chairs, and, in the arts faculty, James Russell and Adam Ferguson had been satisfied and James Balfour had been moved to a sinecure post. The larger context of these moves is discussed in R.B. Sher, *Church and University in the Scottish Enlightenment* (Princeton, 1985), 117–19, 139. See also C.H. Brock, 'The happiness of riches' in Bynum and Porter (n6), 46; Mure (n57), 1, pt II: 262, 267, 278; Hugh Blair to David Hume, 15 April 1764, NLS. Hume Papers formerly held at the Royal Society of Edinburgh. Some sense of the bitter controversy which Cullen's translation provoked can be found in *A Letter from a Citizen of Edinburgh to Doctor Puff [Cullen]* (Edinburgh, 1764). More is apparent in the minutes of the Royal College of Physicians during these years. These feelings had old roots, see Anderson (n53), 9.

89. Donovan, (n65), 181–2; Joseph Black to John Black, 30 June 1766, EUL Gen. 874.5.

90. Fletcher and Brown (n17), 57–9; D.B. Horn MSS, EUL Gen 1824, Box 1, 'Botany', p.19. John Hope to David Skene, 5 and 28 December 1767; 11 April 1768, Aberdeen University Library, David Skene correspondence, MS 38.

91. R. Kerr, *Memoirs of the life, writings and correspondence of William Smellie*, 2 vols, Edinburgh 1811 vol. 1, 261–2.

92. *Medical Commentaries* 4 (1776) 4: Part 1; 99–101 (Editorial comment).

93. R.L. Emerson, 'The Scottish Enlightenment and the end of the Philosophical Society of Edinburgh', *Brit. Jnl for the Hist. of Science*, 21 (1988) 36–48.

94. William Cullen to William Mure, 19 September 1770, Mure (n57), 2:176. Duncan seems to have had testimonials from 'all the members of the medical faculty of Edinburgh, and from other eminent members of the profession'; Chambers (n58), 2:170.

95. Robert Cullen to Adam Smith, 24 June 1761 in *The Correspondence of Adam Smith*, 2nd rev. ed., eds E.C. Mossner and I.S. Ross (Indianapolis), 1987, 76. James Ogilvie, Lord Deskford, to Cullen, 22 January 1764, GUL, Thomson/Cullen 2255/78; Adam Ferguson to Cullen, GUL, ibid, 2255/24; David Hume to Cullen, 21 January 1752 in *The Letters of David Hume*, 2 vols, ed. J.Y.T. Greig (Oxford, 1932), 1:163.

96. Grant (n34), 2:351; Horn (n90), 8.

97. Principal and Professors to Baron Mure, 5 May 1766, Mure (n57), 2:83–4; Thomas Reid tried to interest David or George Skene, Aberdeen MDs, in this post. He believed the Glasgow men would 'be divided, and, consequently, our recommendation, if any is given, will have little weight at Court'. Thomas Reid to David Skene, 18 April 1766, *Thomas Reid: Philosophical Works*, 2 vols, ed. W. Hamilton (Hildesheim, 1967) 1:46. Stevenson had the support of Mure and Lord Loudoun. Alexander Stevenson to the Earl of Loudon, 21 April 1766, Mount Stuart House, Loudoun MSS.

98. See Anderson (n53), 45–6.

99. The story can be followed in the Minutes of the Royal College of Surgeons of Edinburgh, vol.6: 66–151, *passim*; on the quarrel of the two Dundases see L. Naimer and J. Brooke, *The History of Parliament: The House of Commons 1754–1790*, 3 vols (London, 1964), 1: 502–3. R.M. Sunter, *Patronage and Politics in Scotland, 1707–1832* (Edinburgh, 1986), 88–112.

100. Quoted in I.D.L. Clark, 'From Protest to Reaction: The Moderate Regime in the Church of Scotland, 1752–1805' in *Scotland in the Age of*

Improvement, ed. N.T. Phillipson and R. Mitchison (Edinburgh, 1970), 203.

101. Duncan was clearly a supporter of Dundas and his interest until c.1780. Successive volumes of the *Medical Commentaries* were dedicated to William Robertson (1773), the Earl of Kinnoull (1774), William Fullarton of Carstairs (1775, but later probably a Foxite Whig), the Duke of Buccleuch (1776), James Montgomery (1777), Henry Dundas (1779). From that date until the journal ended in 1795 no more dedicatees came from the Dundas camp. Duncan was, however, proud to inform his readers that Cullen had approved of both his and James Gregory's appointments in 1789 and 1790. *Medical Commentaries* 1790, 15: 499.

102. Mackie (n36), 226.

103. Boney (n31), 205–6. The Marquis of Graham to the Masters, 16 March 1790, GUA 58359. In that the Marquis told the professors that they should not petition the Crown for a particular professor because 'Government is always jealous of its Patronage'.

104. In 1788 Stevenson's vote in the election was said to belong to Dundas's friend Sir Adam Ferguson. While the doctor was 'pretty independent', he was also noted as having 'a family and nephews to provide for'. That usually meant siding with the ministry and its friends. *A View of the Political State of Scotland . . . 1788*, ed. C.E. Adam (Edinburgh, 1887), 35; Namier and Brooke (n99), 2: 419–21.

105. George Jardine to Robert Hunter, 25 November 1795, GUL MS Gen 507, Box 1.

106. George Jardine to Robert Hunter, 16 July 1801, GUL MS Gen 505, Box 3.

9

William Cullen's Synopsis Nosologiae Methodicae

ROBERT E. KENDELL

In 1769, when he was 59 years old and at the height of his fame, Cullen published in his *Synopsis Nosologiae Methodicae*, his own comprehensive and elaborate classification of human diseases divided into four classes, nineteen orders and one hundred and thirty two genera. It was widely acclaimed and widely disseminated. The original Latin text ran to at least five editions (1769, 1772, 1780, 1785 and 1792), and several of these were reprinted in Holland, Germany and Italy. After his death English translations were also produced in Springfield, Connecticut in 1793, in Edinburgh in 1800 and in London in 1823. Yet within a generation, the whole elaborate classification was discredited, discarded and forgotten. The purpose of this brief essay is to explain this sequence of events.

The story begins with Thomas Sydenham (1624–89). Unlike his contemporaries, the iatrochemists and iatrophysicists, Sydenham had little time either for the sterile traditions of medical scholarship or for elaborate theories explaining the causes of all diseases. Instead, like Hippocrates, he advocated a detailed study of the actual phenomena of illness. He kept careful notes of his own observations of the patients he attended and it was he who first distinguished between measles and scarlet fever, and between small pox and chicken pox, and who first described rheumatic chorea. He also insisted that each individual disease possessed a uniform set of characteristics, and by implication an independent existence, analogous in every way to that of botanical species:

> Nature, in the production of disease, is uniform and consistent; so much so, that for the same disease in different persons the symptoms are for the most part the same; and the self-same phenomena that you would observe in the sickness of a Socrates you would observe in the sickness of a simpleton.

Indeed, although he never used the term, it is Sydenham to whom we owe the concept of a clinical syndrome, a cluster of associated symptoms and signs with a characteristic tendency to remit, to progress or to recur. In an oft-repeated passage he emphasised that diseases 'were to be reduced to certain and determinate kinds with the same exactness as we see it done by botanic writers in their treatises of plants', and that this could be done by virtue of 'certain distinguishing signs which nature has particularly affixed to every species'. The analogy between diseases and botanical species was explicit and increasingly influential as Sydenham's reputation rose after his death and as detailed taxonomies of animals and plants began to be constructed by naturalists.

Although the Swiss physician, Felix Platter, and the Amsterdam physician, Johnston, had made halting attempts to develop similar classifications of diseases in the seventeenth century, Sydenham's challenge was first wholeheardly accepted by the Montpellier physician François Boissier de Sauvages. Significantly, Boissier de Sauvages (1706–67) had been trained both as a botanist and as a physician. After publishing a small anonymous treatise, *Traité des Classes des Maladies*, in 1731 when he was only 25, and being commended by Boerhaave himself for doing so, he devoted his whole life to the task of elaborating a comprehensive classification of disease. His definitive *Nosologia Methodica Sistens Morborum Classes, Genera et Species, juxta Sydenhami mentem et Botanicorum ordinem* was eventually published in Latin in 1763 and, after his death, in French in 1770–1.

Boissier de Sauvages' classification was quite explicitly modelled on the classification of plants and contained no less than 2,400 species of disease, grouped together in successive stages into genera, orders and finally into ten classes. Nothing so ambitious had ever been attempted before and his tour de force aroused intense interest and inspired a succession of imitators.

The first and most famous of these was the great Swedish botanist Carl von Linné (1707–78), known to posterity by his Latin name Linnaeus. Like Boissier de Sauvages, Linné was both a botanist and a physician. After taking a degree in medicine at Uppsala he spent his formative years as a lecturer in botany studying the vegetation of Lapland and published his *Systema Naturae* in 1735. It was Linnaeus who first enunciated the principles for defining genera and species and introduced the convention of twin names (genus and species) for all species of both animals and plants. His classification of plants was also very influential, because it was based on easily identified features of the plant, and based mainly on flower parts, which tend to remain unchanged during the course of evolution.

Linnaeus read Boissier de Sauvages' original *Traité* in 1735 while he was studying in Holland, and for the next thirty years the two men carried on an extensive correspondence and became close friends, though they never actually met. Linné greatly admired Boissier de

Sauvages' classification of disease and in one of his many letters he said to him:

> You are the only systematician among physicians, you alone have broken the ice and cleared the way. You alone have thrown open the road which blind moles refuse to enter.

In 1738 Linné returned to Sweden to practise as a physician and for a time he held the chair of medicine at Uppsala before exchanging it for the chair of botany. In 1763 he published his own *Genera Morborum*, closely modelled on de Sauvages' classification. Indeed, Linné's classification of diseases was really only a revision and extension of the Montpellier physician's nosology. Most of his genera and species of disease were the same, though they were grouped rather differently, with eleven classes instead of ten and 325 genera instead of 295. The endorsement of so famous a scientist as Linné, however, undoubtedly added to the prestige of Boissier de Sauvages' classification and helped to validate his nosological assumptions and ambitions in the eyes of their contemporaries. In the year following the appearance of Linné's nosology Rudolph Vogel of Göttingen published his *Definitiones Generum Morborum* in which he distinguished 560 genera.

Table 1

The Four Classes and Nineteen Orders of Disease in Cullen's
Nosologia (1769)

Class 1	PYREXIAE	Class 2	NEUROSES
Orders	1. Febres	Orders	1. Comata
	2. Phlegmasiae		2. Adynamiae
	3. Exanthemata		3. Spasmi
	4. Haemorrhagiae		4. Vesaniae
	5. Profluvia		
Class 3	CACHEXIAE	Class 4	LOCALES
Orders	1. Marcores	Orders	1. Dysaesthesiae
	2. Intumescentiae		2. Dyscinesiae
	3. Impetigines		3. Apocenoses
			4. Epischeses
			5. Tumores
			6. Ectopiae
			7. Dialyses

This was the setting in which Cullen's book on the classification of diseases, *Synopsis Nosologiae Methodicae*, was published in 1769. It contained a synopsis of de Sauvages' nosology (1768, emended edition) and the complete nosologies of Linné (1763), Vogel (1764) and Cullen

(1769). Comparison of the four classifications was facilitated by cross references in the text and the general index. The title of Cullen's own classification was *Genera Morborum Praecipua Definita* but it is usually referred to in terms of the general title of the book. Cullen was thoroughly familiar with Linné's classification of plants which he had used in his botany lectures in Glasgow between 1747 and 1750 and he had long been persuaded of the need for a similar classification of diseases. He appreciated the difficulties in producing a satisfactory nosology. Although he praised the attempts which had been made by de Sauvages, Linné and Vogel, he believed that he could improve their achievements significantly. No sooner had Cullen been promoted to the Edinburgh chair of the practice of physic in 1769 than he considered it his duty 'to excite my students to the study of Nosology'. Recognising that this aim might be more easily accomplished by making available to his class the recent continental publications on the subject, he had them printed in juxtaposition to his own nosology in *Synopsis Nosologiae Methodicae*.

The general format and philosophy of Cullen's classification of diseases was identical to those of de Sauvages, Linné and Vogel. It is clear that he attached the same high importance to accurate classification as they had done: 'The distinction of the genera of diseases, the distinction of the species of each, and often even that of the varieties, I hold to be a necessary foundation of every plan of Physic, whether Dogmatical or Empirical.' The detailed structure of his classification was quite different, however. Cullen recognised only four classes of disease – Pyrexiae, Neuroses, Cachexiae and Locales – and only two of these – Pyrexiae and Cachexiae – had been recognised by his predecessors (see Table 1 opposite). These four classes were divided into 19 orders which contained between them 132 genera. In later editions of his work Cullen added a considerable number of species to his classification which he had carefully selected from de Sauvages' nosology. There were, for example, seven species of asthma, five of haemoptysis, four of gonorrhoea and two of nostalgia (simple and complicated).

In 1771 J M B Sagar of Vienna published his *Systema Morborum Symptomaticum* which Cullen included as a fifth methodological nosology in the third edition of *Synopsis Nosologicae Methodicae*. All of these elaborate nosologies were very similar, both in their formal structure and their underlying assumptions, and Boissier de Sauvages was undoubtedly the catalyst. His nosology was the prototype and it was he who had inspired Linné, Vogel, Cullen and Sagar to emulate him. Linné was the most eminent scientist and it was his classification of plants which had inspired Boissier de Sauvages to develop a comparable classification of diseases. Cullen, however, was the most distinguished and influential physician and his reputation as a teacher, and that of the

Edinburgh Medical School of which he was one of the major luminaries, endowed his nosology with considerable influence and prestige, particularly in Britain and America.

Although all these botanical classifications of disease provided medicine, and medical students in particular, with a comprehensive and ordered framework for their discipline, and an aura of scientific respectability, they all had fundamental weaknesses which made their influence shortlived. They had all been inspired, at least indirectly, by Sydenham but they all in varying degrees neglected his injunction that the way forward lay in careful observation and the accurate identification of those regularities of Nature which we now call clinical syndromes. Most of the 2,400 species of diseases which Boissier de Sauvages and the others described were merely symptoms. Indeed, most of their genera were merely symptoms and their individual species of disease no more than lists of the common settings in which a particular symptom was to be found. For example, in Cullen's nosology, trismus, nystagmus, melaena, dyspnoea and aphonia were all dignified with the title of genus, despite the fact that they lacked anything resembling the set of defining characteristics which demarcated Linné's botanical genera. Several of Cullen's genera, like phthisis, rabies, varicella, variola and scarlatina, were certainly genuine syndromes, but most of them had been defined long before, by Sydenham himself or other physicians. They were not Cullen's own creations. For the most part all these elaborate nosologies were simply catalogues of symptoms. Their elaborately tiered structure was based on superficial resemblances or speculative assumptions about aetiology rather than on knowledge of underlying pathology, and it was not long before their pretensions were exposed and their complexity seen to be a handicap rather than a guide to treatment and the understanding of 'proximate causes'.

Perhaps because he was a more thoughtful and more experienced physician, Cullen seems to have had more insight into the limitations of his classification than most of the other 'botanical nosologists'. He distinguishes three different aspects of nosology – the characterisation and definition of individual diseases, the provision of suitable names, and the arrangement of individual species of disease into genera, classes and orders. He made it clear that he considered the first of these the most important, and that he had doubts about the validity of his classes and orders: 'By nature, species only are given: the formation of genera is the production of the human mind. . . . I have, with others, endeavoured to form classes and orders; but for the accuracy of these, I would by no means vouch.' He also omitted about forty of the diseases he recognised from his classification, admitting candidly that 'I had no clear or accurate knowledge of them, or could not work them into any part of my system.'

The popularisation of dissection of the cadaver in France and Italy towards the end of the eighteenth century led to a growing appreciation of the role of pathological anatomy in the causation of disease. What determined prognosis and the possibilities for treatment was whether or not the patient had gall stones, or a cirrhotic liver, or a strangulated loop of bowel, not simply whether he was suffering from icterus or ileus. Morgagni's seminal work *De Sedibus et Causis Morborum per Anatomen Indagatis* had been published in 1761, two years before the definitive version of Boissier de Sauvages' *Nosologia* and eight years before Cullen's *Synopsis*. Its immediate impact on medical thinking was less dramatic than that of the *Nosologia*, but as postmortem dissection slowly became a routine procedure in the medical schools of continental Europe it became increasingly clear that pathology was going to be the science of the future rather than botany, and that until the true causes of disease were better understood elaborate classifications served little purpose. Cullen himself seems to have been aware of the importance of postmortem dissection. In a clinical lecture to his students in 1772 he observed that:

> It is not improperly said that the earth hides the faults of the physician. If every patient that dies was opened, as ours has been, it would but too often discover the frivolity of our conjectures and practice . . . with regard to the present case I might go back to consider the symptoms, and from them endeavour to account for my own ignorance; but I choose rather to acknowledge my mistakes, and to consider the case on the footing which we have now learned from dissection.

He expressed similar sentiments in the preface to the 1784 edition of his *First Lines of the Practice of Physic*, observing that 'in establishing a proper pathology, there is nothing that has been of more service than the Dissection of morbid bodies' and paying tribute to 'the great and valuable work of the illustrious Morgagni'. However, as Risse (1986) has shown, postmortem dissection was rarely performed in Edinburgh, or indeed elsewhere in Britain, in the eighteenth century and morbid anatomy had little influence on Cullen's nosology. This was partly because the young adults who constituted the bulk of the patients admitted to the Edinburgh Royal Infirmary rarely died in hospital, because relatives were reluctant to give permission for autopsies, and because the hospital's managers were insistent that unauthorised dissections were not to be countenanced. It also seems to have been the case that, despite the admirable sentiments expressed in his 1772 lecture, Cullen and his fellow physicians generally took little interest in postmortem examinations, and also used them mainly to illustrate the diagnoses they had previously made on clinical grounds rather than to determine the true diagnosis and the underlying pathology. Indeed,

Cullen argued at times that morbid anatomy ought not to influence diagnosis and nosology because its findings were not 'directly evident, and only such marks ought to be employed as are evident'. The Edinburgh surgeons were more enlightened. They performed more and more thorough postmortems and learnt more from them. Cullen realised, of course, that a classification of disease which was not based on an accurate identification of 'proximate causes' was of little value. He maintained, however, that 'I have generally endeavoured to obviate the consequences of this, by proving, that the proximate causes which I have assigned are true, in fact, as well as deductions from any reasoning that I may seem to have employed'. Unfortunately, subsequent events proved that he was mistaken.

Although there seems to be little doubt that Cullen's students, and many of his contemporaries, found his classification valuable and regarded it as an important scientific advance, he and his fellow botanical nosologists were not without contemporary critics. Sir John Pringle made it clear that he regarded the construction of nosologies as 'a frivolous and unattainable pursuit' and Plocquet, Mason Good and Young were all very critical of many aspects of Cullen's classification. They criticised him for confusing genera and species and indeed Cullen himself openly admitted that no less than a hundred of the genera of disease described in the first (1769) edition of his *Nosologia* 'are properly species, and admit of no farther division'. Good and Young also derided him for not knowing where to put his *omissi* (the forty diseases he left unclassified), for parts of his nomenclature and for many aspects of the detailed structure of his nosology. Even his admiring pupil, Benjamin Rush, could not resist mocking Cullen's predilection for useless distinctions by dividing phobias into eighteen species, including rum phobia ('a very rare disease'), want phobia ('confined chiefly to old people') and church phobia ('endemic in the city of Philadelphia') (Rush, 1812).

After Cullen's death and the cataclysmic events of the French revolution and the Napoleonic wars, Cullen's nosology, like those of de Sauvages, Linné, Vogel, Sagar and the Dublin physician Macbride, was not so much criticised as ignored and forgotten. For by then it was apparent to most physicians that complicated tiered classifications of disease served little purpose. They were a hindrance rather than a help both to therapeutics and to the search for 'proximate causes' and the seductive analogy with botanical species was an illusion.

With hindsight we can also appreciate that the ambitions and pretensions of the botanical nosologists were not thwarted merely by their profound ignorance of aetiology. Two hundred years later when vastly more is known about the aetiology and pathogenesis of human diseases, we still do not find it appropriate to construct elaborately tiered classifications of disease, or to use the terminology of natural history. The groupings of disease we currently recognise are groupings of convenience, corresponding to the spheres of influence of individual medical specialties rather than to what we take to be fundamental biological distinctions. Cerebrovascular disease is classified with diseases of the central nervous system, not with peripheral vascular disease or coronary artery disease, because its consequences are treated by neurologists and neurosurgeons; and Alzheimer's disease and most other dementias are classified as mental disorders rather than neurological disorders because they are generally treated by psychiatrists. But although Cullen and his fellow nosologists were misguided in assuming that medicine would benefit from an elaborately tiered classification of diseases, and wrong to assume that every category, of animal or plant, disease or mineral, must be dignified with both a specific and a generic name, Cullen himself was absolutely right to insist on the importance of accurately identifying and defining individual diseases. That task is as important today as it was in the eighteenth century, and it is greatly to Cullen's credit that he realised more clearly that any of the other nosologists of his day where the true priorities of medicine should lie.

The most interesting and novel part of Cullen's nosology was the second of his four classes of disease, the Neuroses, or Nervous Diseases. Neurosis was a new term which Cullen coined to describe 'All those preternatural affections of sense or motion which are without pyrexia . . . and all those which do not depend upon a topical affection of organs, but upon a more general affection of the nervous system, and of those powers of the system upon which sense and motion more especially depend.' The term embraced four orders of disease – *Comata* (including apoplexy); *Adynamiae* (including hypochondriasis, dyspepsia, syncope and chlorosis); *Spasmi* (including convulsions and hysteria, but also dyspnoea, diabetes, pertussis, tetanus, colic and cholera); and *Vesaniae* (an old Roman term for insanity, revived by Boissier de Sauvages). The complete text of the Neuroses section in an early English translation of Cullen's nosology is reproduced in an appendix, pp. 226–33. It well illustrates both the complexity and the lack of detailed description of individual species of disease of the classification as a whole. Clearly Neuroses embraced a large part of medicine, including, but by no means restricted to, what we now regard as neurological and psychiatric disorders.

The rationale for this grouping derived from Cullen's belief that the normal functioning of the body was dependent on 'nervous energy' derived from the nervous system. This was a recurring theme in his teaching and the main thesis of his four volume textbook, *First Lines of the Practice of Physic*, published between 1777 and 1784. Like many other physicians before and since, Cullen gradually convinced himself

that excesses or deficiencies, local or general, of the hypothetical
influence which interested him most, 'nervous energy', were the root
cause of most disease. His interest in the nervous system and its
pathology was partly derived from the neuroanatomical discoveries of
the seventeenth-century English physician Thomas Willis (1622–75) and
partly from the work of Boerhaave's pupil, Haller (1708–77). Haller,
who is sometimes referred to as the father of physiology, had conducted
an ingenious series of experiments on nervous conduction, muscle
contraction and afferent sensation in which he demonstrated that nerves
possessed intrinsic sensibility and that muscle had an intrinsic irritability, the *vis insita*, quite independent of the influence of volition.

Cullen was also influenced both by George Cheyne (1671–1743) and
by his distinguished contemporary and predecessor in the chair of
the Institutes of Medicine in Edinburgh, Robert Whytt (1714–66).
Cheyne's treatise on *The English Malady* (1733) had popularised the
concept of 'Nervous Diseases' a generation before. He wrote from
personal experience of depression and regarded his nervous disease as
'the most deplorable, and beyond comparison the worst . . . of all the
Miseries that afflict Human Life'. He was also well aware that they were
'under some Kind of Disgrace and Imputation, in the Opinion of the
Vulgar and Unlearned' and was therefore at pains to emphasise that
nervous diseases mainly affected people 'of the liveliest and quickest
natural Parts . . . whose Genius is most keen and penetrating', and that
they 'make almost one third of the complaints of the people of condition
in England'. Whytt's interest in nervous disorders was less personal and
more scholarly and his monograph entitled *Observations on the Nature,
Causes, and Cure of those Disorders which have been commonly called
Nervous, Hypochondriacal or Hysteric*, published in 1765, was widely
read.

After commenting rather ruefully that 'Physicians have bestowed the
character of nervous on all those disorders whose nature and causes they
were ignorant of' Whytt went on to observe that:

> All diseases may, in some sense, be called affections of the nervous
> system, because, in almost every disease, the nerves are more or
> less hurt; and, in consequence of this, various sensations, motions,
> and changes, are produced in the body. However, those disorders
> may, peculiarly, deserve the name of nervous, which, on account of
> an unusual delicacy, or unnatural state of the nerves, are produced
> by causes, which, in people of a sound constitution, would either
> have no such effects, or at least in a much less degree.

Whytt's Nervous Disorders were, however, more restricted in scope
that Cullen's Neuroses, for he only recognised three varieties – hysteria,
hypochondriasis and those, like palpitations, faintings and convulsive
fits, which he called 'simply nervous'.

Although Cullen's *Nosology* did not long survive his death and although his theory that all life was a manifestation of 'nervous energy' and most disease a form of nervous disorder had scant empirical justification, he did succeed in focusing the interest of his contemporaries and pupils on the nervous system rather than the heart and vascular system, which had held pride of place for both Harvey and Boerhaave. In a sense, therefore, he can claim to be the father of neuropathology and neurology. And his term Neurosis survived.

For Cullen, Neuroses had been 'affections of sense or motion which are without pyrexia'. For his nineteenth-century successors they became functional disorders of the nervous system with no known structural pathology. The great French alienist Pinel (1745–1826) was probably instrumental in ensuring the survival of the term for he translated Cullen's textbook into French and made the Neuroses the centrepiece of his own classification. Pinel himself distinguished five categories of neurosis (Neuroses of the senses; of cerebral function; of locomotion; of nutrition; and of sexual function: Reynold, 1990). Although subsequent developments in morbid anatomy and histology progressively reduced the range of functional (i.e. without structural pathology) disorders of the nervous system the term survived to the closing years of the nineteenth century when it was adopted and immortalised by Sigmund Freud and the school of psychoanalysis he created. Freud initially distinguished between psychoneuroses (hysteria and obsessive compulsive neurosis) which were due to a nervous excitation which was psychic in origin and actual neuroses (neurasthenia and anxiety neurosis) which were caused by an excess or deficiency of 'somatic excitation'. These 'actual neuroses' were virtually a reincarnation of Cullen's original concept, for Freud's libido was little more than a sexualised form of Cullen's 'nervous energy' and he regarded his actual neuroses as direct consequences of the accumulation or dissipation of libido. The distinction between actual and psychoneuroses did not survive beyond the 1930s but neurosis itself is still one of the great words of psychiatry. Like most psychiatric concepts it has changed its original meaning out of all recognition and is now much criticised for its vagueness and the untenable psychodynamic assumptions still trailing in its wake. A proposal by the American Psychiatric Association in 1980 to drop the term from its nomenclature caused such dismay and indignation that the young Turks who wished to bury it were forced to compromise. So neurosis still survives, albeit somewhat precariously, and with it our link with an outstanding clinician and an inspiring and influential teacher.

Bibliography

Cheyne, G. (1733) *The English Malady: or, A Treatise of Nervous Diseases of all Kinds, as Spleen, Vapours, Lowness of Spirits, Hypochondriacal and Hysterical Distempers* (Strahan & Leake: London).

Cullen, W. 1777–84 *First Lines of the Practice of Physic* (Murray, Creech, Elliot and Cadell: Edinburgh and London, 4 vols, 1796 edition).

Cullen, W. (1780) *Synopsis Nosologiae Methodicae* (2 vols, 3rd Edn., Creech: Edinburgh).

Cullen, W. (1827) *The Works of William Cullen, MD* (2 vols, edited by J. Thomson, Blackwood: Edinburgh).

Freud, S. (1922) *Introductory Lectures on Psychoanalysis* (George Allen & Unwin: London).

Hunter, R. & Macalpine, I. (1963) *Three Hundred Years of Psychiatry* (Oxford University Press: London).

Kendell, R.E. (1975) *The Role of Diagnosis in Psychiatry* (Blackwell: Oxford).

Knoff, W.F. (1970) 'A history of the concept of neurosis, with a memoir of William Cullen', *American Journal of Psychiatry* **127**, 80–4.

McGirr, E.M. (1990) *Cullen in context*, Stevenson Lecture, University of Glasgow, 14th February 1990.

Reynolds, E.H. (1990) 'Structure and function in neurology and psychiatry', *British Journal of Psychiatry* **157**, 481–90.

Risse, G.B. (1986) *Hospital life in Enlightenment Scotland* (Cambridge University Press: Cambridge).

Rush, B. (1812) *Medical Inquiries and Observations upon the Diseases of the Mind* (Kimber and Richardson: Philadelphia).

Stott, R. (1987) 'Health and virtue: or how to keep out of harm's way. Lectures on pathology and therapeutics by William Cullen c.1770', *Medical History* **31**, 123–42.

Thomson, J. (1859) *An Account of the Life, Lectures and Writings of William Cullen, MD* (2 vols, vol. 1 first published 1832; Blackwood: Edinburgh).

Whytt, R. (1765) *Observations on the nature, causes and cure of those disorders which have been called nervous, hypochondriac, or hysteric, to which are prefixed some remarks on the sympathy of the nerves* (Becket & Du Hondt: Edinburgh).

APPENDIX – CULLEN'S CLASSIFICATION OF NEUROSES

From *Synopsis and nosology, being an arrangement and definition of diseases by William Cullen, MD. The second edition, translated from Latin to English* (Published 1793; Edward Gray: Springfield, Connecticut.)

Class II. NEUROSES. An injury of the sense and motion, without an Idiopathic Pyrexia or any local affection.

Order I. COMATA. A dimunition of voluntary motion, with sleep, or a deprivation of the senses.

Genus 42. Apoplexia. Almost all voluntary motion diminished, with sleep more or less profound; the motion of the heart and arteries remaining.

The Idiopathic Species are:

1. Apoplexia (sanguinea) with symptoms of universal plethora, especially of the head.
2. Apoplexia (serosa) with a lucophlegmasia over the whole body, especially in old people.

3. Apoplexia (Hydrocephalica) coming on by degrees, affecting infants, or those below the age of puberty first with lassitude, a slight fever and pain of the head, then with slowness of the pulse, dilatation of the pupil of the Eye, and drowsiness.

4. Apoplexia (atrabiliaria) taking place in those of a Melancholic constitution.

5. Apoplexia (traumatica) from some external injury mechanically applied to the head.

6. Apoplexia (venenata) from powerful sedatives taken internally or applied externally.

7. Apoplexia (mentalis) from a passion of the mind.

8. Apoplexia (Cataleptica) in the contractile muscles, with immobility of the limbs by external force.

9. Apoplexia (suffocata) from some external suffocating power.

The Apoplexy is frequently symptomatic.

1. Of an intermittent fever.	6. Epilepsy
2. Continued fever.	7. Podagra.
3. Phlegmasiae.	8. Worms.
4. Exanthema.	9. Ischuria.
5. Hysteria.	10. Scurvys.

Genus 43. Paralysis. Only some of the voluntary motions diminished, frequently with sleep.

The Idiopathic Species are.

1. Paralysis (partialis) of some particular muscles only.

2. Paralysis, (hemiplegia) of one side of the body. Vary according to the constitution of the body.

a. Hemiplegia in a plethoric habit.

b. In a leucophlegmatic habit.

3. Paralysis (paraplegia) of one half of the body taken transversly.

4. Paralysis (venenata) from sedative powers applied either externally or internally.

II. Species are.

A. Symptoms either of an asthenia or palsy, tremor, an alternate motion of a limb by frequent strokes and intervals.

The Species are.

1. Asthenia.

2. Paralytic.

3. Convulsive.

Order II. ADYNAMIAE. A diminution of the involuntary motions, whether vital or natural.

Genus 44. Syncope, a dimunition or even a total stoppage, of the motion of the heart for a little.

I. Idiopathic.

1. Syncope (cardiaca) returning frequently without any manifest cause, with violent palpatations of the heart, during the intervals from a fault of the heart or neighbouring vessels.
2. Syncope (occasionalis) arising from some evident cause, from an affection of the whole system.

II. Symptomatic, or symptoms of disease, either of the whole system, or of other parts besides the heart.

Genus 45. Dyspepsia. Anorexia, nausea, vomiting, inflation, belching, rumination, cardialgia, gastrodynia, more or fewer of those symptoms at least concuring, for the most with a constipation of the belly, and without any other diseases either of the stomach itself, or of other parts.

I. Idiopathic.

II. Symptomatic.
1. From a disease of the stomach itself.
2. From a disease of other parts, or of the whole body.

Genus 46. Hypochondriasis, dyspepsia, with langour, sadness and fear without any adequate causes, in a melancholic temperament.

Genus 47. Chlorosis. Dyspepsia, or a desire of something not used as food, a pale or discoloured complexion. The veins not well filled, a soft tumour of the whole body, asthenia, palpitation, suppression of the menses.

Order III. SPASMI. Irregular motions of the muscles or muscular fibres.

Sect. I. *In the animal functions.*

Genus 48. Tetanus. A spastic rigidity of almost the whole body. Varying according to the remote cause as it arises either from something internal, from cold, or from a wound. It varies likewise, from whatever cause it arises according to the part of the body affected.

Genus 49. Trismus. As spastic rigidity of the lower jaw. The Species are.

1. Trismus (nascentium) seizing infants under two months old.

2. Trismus (traumaticus) seizing people of all ages either from wound or cold.

Genus 50. Convulsio, an irregular clonic contraction of the muscles without sleep.

1. Idiopathic.   2. Symptomatic.

Genus 51. Chorea. Attacking those who have not yet arrived at puberty, most commonly within the 10th or 14th year, with convulsive motions for the most part of one side, in attempting the voluntary motions of the hands and arms, resembling the gesticulations of mountebanks, in walking rather dragging one of their feet after them, than lifting it.

Genus 52. Raphania. A spastic contraction of the joints, with convulsive agitations and most violent periodical pain.

Genus 53. Epilepsia. A convulsion of the muscles, with sleep.

The Idiopathic Species are.

1. Epilepsia (cerebralis) suddenly attacking without any manifest cause, without any sense of uneasiness preceeding, excepting perhaps a slight vertigo or Scotoma.
2. Epilepsia (Sympathica) without any manifest cause, but preceeded by the sensation of a kind of air rising from a certain part of the body towards the head.
3. Epilepsia (occasionalis) arising from a manifest irritation and ceasing on the removal of that irritation. Varying according to the difference of the irritating matter, and thus it may arise.
From injuries of the head, pain, worms, poison, from the repulsion of the itch, or an effusion of any other acrid humor, from crudities in the stomach, from passions of the mind, from an immoderate haemorrhage, or from debility.

Sect. II. *In the vital functions.*

A. In the action of the heart.

Genus 54. Palpitatio. A violent and irregular motion of the heart.

B. In the action of the Lungs.

Genus 55. Asthma. A difficulty of breathing, returning by intervals, with a sense of straitness in the breast, and a noisy respiration with hissing; in the beginning of the paroxysm there is either no cough at all, or coughing is difficult, but towards the end the cough becomes free, frequently with a copious spitting of mucus.

The Idiopathic Species are.

1. Asthma (spontaneum) without any manifest cause or other concomitant disease.
2. Asthma (exanthematicum) from the repulsion of the Itch or acrid effusion.
3. Asthma (plethoricum) from the suppression of some customary sanguineous evacuation or from a spontaneous plethora.
Genus 56. Dyspnoea. A continual difficulty of breathing, without any sense of straitness, but rather of fullness and infraction in the breast, a frequent cough throughout the whole course of the disease.

The Idiopathic species are.

1. Dyspnoea (catarrhalis) with a frequent cough, bringing up plenty of viscid mucus.
2. Dyspnoea. (sicca) with a cough, for the most part dry.
3. Dyspnoea. (aerea) increased by the least change of weather.
4. Dyspnoea. (terrea) bringing up with the cough an earthy or calculous matter.
5. Dyspnoea. (aquosa) with scanty urine and oedematous fat, without any signs of an Hydrothorax.
6. Dyspnoea. (pinguedinosa) in very fat people.
7. Dyspnoea. (thoracica) from an injury done to the parts surrounding the thorax or from some bad conformation of them.
8. Dyspnoea. (extrinseca) from evident external causes.

The symptomatic Species of dyspnoea are symptoms.

1. Of diseases of the heart or large vessels.
2. Of swellings in the abdomen.
3. Of various diseases.

Genus 57. Pertussis. A contagious disease, convulsive strangulating cough, reiterated with noisy inspiration, frequent vomiting.

Sect. II. *In the natural functions.*

Genus 58. Pyrosis. A burning pain in the epigastrium with plenty of aqueous humour, for the most part insipid, but sometimes acrids belchings up.

Genus 59. Colica. Pain of the belly, especially twisting round the navel, vomiting, a constipation. The Idiopathic Species are.

1. Colica (spasmodica) with retraction of the navel, and spasms of the abdominal muscles. Varying by reason of some symptoms super-added. Hence,
a. Colica, with vomiting of excrements, or of matters injected by the anus.
b. Colica, with inflammation supervening.

2. Colica (pictonum) preceded by a sense of weight or uneasiness in the belly, especially about the navel, then comes on the colic pain, at first slight and interrupted, chiefly augmented after meals, at length more severe and almost continual, with pain of the arms and back, at last ending in a Palsy. Varying according to the nature of the remote cause, and hence,
a. From metallic poison.
b. From acids taken inwardly.
c. From cold.
d. From a contusion of the back.
3. Colica (stercorea) in people subject to costiveness.
4. Colica (accidentalis) from acrid matter taken internally.
5. Colica (meconialis) in new-born children from a retention of the meconium.

6. Colica (callosa) with a sensation of stricture in some part of the intestines and frequently of a collection of flatus with some pain before the constricted part, which flatus also passing through the part where the stricture is felt gradually vanishes. The belly slow, and at last passing only a few liquid faeces.

7. Colica (calculosa) with a fixed hardness in some part of the abdomen, and calculi sometimes passing by the anus.

Genus 60. Cholera. A vomiting of bilious matter, and likewise a frequent excretion of the same by stool, anxiety, gripes, spasm in the calves of the legs.

I.Idiopathic.

1. Cholera, (spontanea) arising in a warm season without any manifest cause.

2. Cholera. (accidentalis) from acrid matters taken internally.

II. Symptomatic.

Genus 61. Diarrhoea. Frequent stools, the disease not infectious, no primary pyrexia.

I. Idiopathic.

1. Diarrhoea (crapulosa) in which the excrements are voided in greater quantity than naturally.

2. Diarrhoea (biliosa) in which yellow faeces are voided in great quantity.

3. Diarrhoea (mucosa) in which either from acrid substances taken inwardly, or from cold, especially applied to the feet; a great quantity is voided.

4. Diarrhoea (coeliaca) in which a milky humour of the nature of chyle is passed.

5. Diarrhoea (lienteria) in which the aliments are discharged with little alteration soon after eating.

6. Diarrhoea (hepatirrhoea) in which a bloody serous matter is discharged without pain.

II.Symptomatic.

Genus 62. Diabetes. A chronical profusion of urine, for the most part preternatural and in immoderate quantity.

I. Idiopathic.

I. Diabetes (mellitus) with urine of the smell, colour, and flavour of honey.

II. Diabetes (insipidus) with limpid, but not sweet urine.

II. Symptomatic.

Genus 63. Hysteria. Rumbling of the bowels; a sensation of a globe turning itself in the belly, ascending to the stomach; sleep; convulsions; a great quantity of limpid urine; the mind involuntary fickle and mutable. The following are by Sauvages reckoned distinct Idiopathic Species, but by Dr Cullen, only varieties of the same Species.

A. From a retention of the menses.
B. From a menorrhagia (cruenta).
C. From a menorrhagia serosa or flour albus.
D. From an obstruction of the viscera.
E. From a fault of the stomach.
F. From too great Salacity.

Genus 64. Hydrophobia. A dislike and horror at every kind of drink, as occasioning a convulsion of the pharynx, induced for the most part, by the bite of a mad animal.

The Species are.

I. Hydrophobia (rabiosa) with a desire of biting the by-standers, occasioned by the bite of a mad animal.
II. Hydrophobia (simplex) without madness, or any desire of biting.

Order IV. VESANIAE. Disorders of the judgment without any pyrexia or coma.

Genus 65. Amentia. An imbecility of judgment, by which people do not perceive, or do not remember the relations of things.

The Species are.

I. Amentia. (congenita) continuing from a person's birth.
II. Amentia. (senilis) from the diminution of the perceptions and memory through extreme old age.
III. Amentia. (acquisita) occurring in people formerly of a sound mind, from evident external causes.

Genus 66. Melancholia. A partial madness, without dyspepsia. Varying according to the different subjects concerning which the person raves. And thus is,

1. With an Imagination in the patient concerning his body being in a dangerous condition, from slight causes, or that his affairs are in a desperate state.
2. With an Imagination concerning a prosperous state of affairs.
3. With violent love, without satyriasis or nymphomania.
4. With a superstitious fear of a future state.
5. With an aversion from motion and all the offices of life.
6. With restlessness and an impatience of any situation whatever.
7. With a weariness of life.
8. With a deception concerning the nature of the patients Species.

The Doctor reckons that there is no such disease as that called Daemonomania, and that the diseases mentioned by Sauvages under that title are either.

1. Species of melancholy or mania.
2. Disease falsely ascribed by spectators to the influence of an evil spirit.
3. Disease entirely feigned.
4. Disease partly true and partly feigned.

Genus 67. Mania. Universal madness.

1. Mania (mentalis) arising entirely from passions of the mind.
2. Mania (corporea) from an evident disease of the body.

Varying according to the different disease of the body.

3. Mania (obscura) without any passion of the mind or evident disease of the body preceeding.

The symptomatic Species of mania are.

1. Paraphrosyne from poisons.
2. Paraphrosyne from passion.
3. Paraphrosyne febrilis.

Genus 68. Oneirodynia. A violent and troublesome imagination in time of sleep.

1. Oneirodynia (activa) exciting to waking and various motions.
2. Oneirodynia (gravans) from a sense of some incumbent weight and pressing the breast especially.

10

Cullen's influence on American medicine

JOHN M. O'DONNELL

My esteemed colleagues and gracious hosts, I am honoured to be among you and bring you the warmest regards from the College of Physicians of Philadelphia, a century younger than the Royal College, founded by Edinburgh graduates, and – two centuries later – still edified by your continuing accomplishments, including this impressive bicentenary celebration.

We are told that when a copy of the Magna Carta arrived in Washington, DC, during the bicentennial celebration of the United States in 1976, it was displayed in a sealed capsule. A British Embassy spokesman explained (and I quote): 'It is breathing the air of the British Museum, so it will be comfortable and not suffer culture shock'. Arriving quite unsealed, I have suffered only cultural stimulation in this exhilarating, fair city, with its great University. It is my hope that you will not be shocked when it becomes apparent that it must have been only kindness and the demands of brevity that persuaded the symposium's organisers to advertise 'a distinguished panel of Cullen scholars' rather than the lengthier accuracy: 'a distinguished panel of Cullen scholars and the director of the College of Physicians of Philadelphia'.

Undeterred, I begin by quoting one of my favourite Americans, the philosopher William James, as he delivered at the beginning of this century at the University of Edinburgh the introductory talk to the Gifford Lectures on Natural Religion, which we know better as the book entitled *The Varieties of Religious Experience*:

> It is with no small amount of trepidation that I take my place behind this desk, and face this learned audience. To us Americans, the experience of receiving instruction from the living voice . . . of European scholars is very familiar . . . It seems the natural thing for us to listen whilst the Europeans talk. The contrary habit, of talking whilst the Europeans listen, we have not yet acquired; and in him who . . . makes the adventure it begets a certain sense of apology being due for so presumptuous an act. Particularly must

this be the case on a soil as sacred to the American imagination as that of Edinburgh.[1]

Doubly so, I would add, when we are talking about the American medical imagination, for, to a determining extent in the last half of the eighteenth century, the ideal images of medical education and organisation held by most influential Americans were formed on Scottish soil and at a time when William Cullen's influence was at its height.

To speak of Cullen's influence as though it were a single stream flowing into a great lake of American medicine would be a metaphorical mistake that would ultimately depreciate Cullen's impact. Instead I should like to write Cullen larger and American medicine smaller. By that I mean that his influence was direct, and indirect, and multifaceted. Cullen was moisture absorbed into many clouds and mixed with other elements and released at various times over different parts of America's intellectual and institutional terrain. His influence was not a steady stream; it was rain. It was larger than his own professional life.

By writing American medicine smaller, I mean to pursue unabashedly a course of enlightened parochialism and talk about Philadelphia medicine. Four decades of historical scholarship have taught us to avoid the pitfall of assuming that the medicine practised in provincial capitals bears much resemblance to medicine practised in the hinterlands.[2] To speak of eighteenth-century Philadelphia medicine and of American medicine is to describe two things. Nevertheless, it was in Philadelphia and largely, though not exclusively, through Philadelphia that Cullen's influence and the influence of Scottish medicine generally were most manifest.

The preconditions accounting for that fact are, of course, social, economic and cultural. Influence involves scale. And while one of Cullen's American students wrote home in 1764 that 'it must certainly make him [Cullen] very happy . . . to see so many even from the Wilds of America crouding his lectures,'[3] the fact remains that Philadelphia must be seen as a provincial centre in a great Atlantic civilisation, rather than a wilderness outpost (Benjamin Franklin's squirrel hats notwithstanding). The successful utilisation of ideas, imitation of institutions, and emulation of careers require similar socioeconomic ecologies. On the eve of the American Revolution (if I may be allowed to call it that, coming from a different historiographic tradition), the population of greater Philadelphia was about 40,000, slightly larger than that of Edinburgh or Dublin. Thus, Philadelphia, the largest city in America and, with the Revolution, the seat of government until the turn of the century, was probably the second largest metropolis in the British Empire. By mid-century, then, Philadelphia, like any contemporary city of comparable size, had accumulated the wealth to create medical institutions and the poverty to catalyse medical initiative. The concen-

tration of population created unprecedented medical demands; the
limitations of medical science intensified the reality as well as the
perception that these demands were not being met; and the ensuing
competition among 'regular' physicians, 'irregular' and sectarian practitioners in the absence of much valid therapy prompted individual
doctors to feel the need for mutual support. They began to take steps
toward establishing societies. They were beginning to professionalise,
even without the help of twentieth century sociologists to tell them how.
The most ambitious, financially capable, and well connected men
went abroad to seek substantive education as well as imposing credentials. A handful of would-be elites sought also to institutionalise
domestically the patterns of medical organisation found in Europe. In
an imitation of institutions encountered elsewhere, Philadelphia's finest
physicians saw their only hope for the advancement of their professional
careers and the progress of American medicine. That it is difficult for us
– as it must have been virtually impossible for them – to discern the
difference between the two is testimony to their achievement. Quite
self-consciously, these gentlemen attempted to make Philadelphia, in
Chief Justice William Allen's apt phrase, 'the Edinburgh of America.'[4]

This intention was not suddenly realised and enacted. As the Royal
College's own Professor Ronald Girdwood has reminded us, Scotland
has had an influence on North American medicine since the early
seventeenth-century. Several Philadelphians had sought medical
instruction there prior to the middle of the eighteenth century. Certainly, there were other places to go: Leiden, Paris, London, Rheims.
And surely other reasons; a grand tour of the Continent rounded out
not only the doctor but also the gentleman. Nevertheless, several
geographical, social and cultural conditions conspired to make Edinburgh Philadelphia's medical Mecca. Britain was, after all, the mother
country; language was not a barrier; Edinburgh was close to London
and, after 1750, as Richard Shryock points out, London had an ample
supply of what physicians so poetically call 'clinical material.'[5] Philadelphia medicine was largely Quaker medicine (leading, of course, to the
jocular comment occasionally heard today that 'Some of my best
doctors are Friends'), and Edinburgh's moral and political atmosphere
was more auspicious to Quaker fathers than that of London or,
certainly, of Paris. Moreover, as we know, while one would obtain a
first-rate education at Edinburgh, it was also notoriously easy to get a
degree there. In fact, at least one American student signed a petition
protesting what was perceived to be a lowering of standards that the
signatories felt devalued their credentials. Adam Smith wrote quite
plainly to Cullen about the competitive advantages to the Scottish
universities of exploiting the market for international students.[6] In the
last half of the eighteenth century, over one hundred Americans

received their medical degrees from the University of Edinburgh. Many more had studied there. The Scottish medical influence on America was predominantly the influence of its system of medical education and patterns of medical association, two aspects of Scottish medicine which Cullen decisively affected.

The connections between educational systems are unmistakable. When the Medical School of the College of Philadelphia (as the University of Pennsylvania was then called) was founded in 1765, its first six professors – John Morgan, William Shippen, Jr., Adam Kuhn, Benjamin Rush, Philip Syng Physick, and Casper Wistar – had all received their medical degrees from the University of Edinburgh. With respect to professional organisations, one American association, the structure and functions of which have deep roots in the Scottish experiences of many of its founding members, is the College of Physicians of Philadelphia, founded in 1787. At the risk of turning enlightened parochialism shallow, allow me to exposit Cullen's influence upon Philadelphia medicine by illustrating his – and Edinburgh's – connection to the College's founders.

Table 1

THE FOUNDERS OF
THE COLLEGE OF PHYSICIANS OF PHILADELPHIA
1787

SENIOR FELLOWS

John Redman, President
John Jones, Vice-President
James Hutchinson, Secretary
Gerardus Clarkson, Treasurer
William Shippen, Jr., Censor
John Morgan, Censor
Benjamin Rush, Censor
Adam Kuhn, Censor
Samuel Duffield
Thomas Parke
George Glentworth
Abraham Chovet

JUNIOR FELLOWS

Robert Harris	Benjamin Duffield
John Foulke	James Hall
Andrew Ross	William Currie
John Carson	William W. Smith
Samuel P. Griffitts	John Morris
Benjamin Say	William Clarkson

Table 2

FOUNDING MEMBERS OF
COLLEGE OF PHYSICIANS OF PHILADELPHIA IN EDINBURGH
(1752–84)

	At Edinburgh	Degree from Edinburgh	Other European Training
John Jones (1729–91)	1752–3(?)	No	Yes
John Morgan (1735–89)	1761–3	Yes	Yes
George Glentworth (1735–92)	1758–9	No	Yes
William Shippen, Jr (1736–1808)	1760–1	Yes	Yes
Adam Kuhn (1741–1817)	1765–7	Yes	Yes
Benjamin Rush (1745–1813)	1766–8	Yes	Yes
Thomas Parke (1749–1835)	1771–2	No	Yes
Benjamin Duffield (1753–99)	1773–4	No	No
Samuel Griffitts (1759–1826)	1783–4	No	Yes

The twenty-four founding members of the College shown in Table 1 comprised about half of Philadelphia's practising physicians, but they were the most respected and best known men. Half of the founding members received formal training abroad, including all but one of the senior fellows.[7] One third of the entire group received medical schooling at Edinburgh (where four obtained the MD degree: Table 2). Six of the twelve senior fellows were students of Cullen – Morgan, Glentworth, Shippen, Kuhn, Rush and Parke.

The exclusive medical society played an essential role in the organisation of medicine in the last quarter of the eighteenth century on both continents. Medicine must straddle the worlds of detached learning and interested art, and the physician must cultivate the images of scholar and technician. Medical societies, as James H. Cassedy has pointed out, are the vehicles within which resolution of these ambiguities is attempted. Such organisations are intermediate between the medical school and the individual doctor's office. Given the conflicts among eighteenth century physicians and between doctors and patients caused by the invalidity of most therapies, medical societies succeeded when small groups of physicians separated themselves from other practitioners, formed exclusive societies, attempted to achieve or enforce consensus on therapies, published transactions, consulted among themselves, and attempted to control appointments to medical college faculties. These exclusive societies typically were composed of the best educated physicians who tended to treat the best educated clientele.[8] Like their patients, therefore, they tended to be relatively affluent. They did not hesitate to use their wealth as capital to improve local institutions or to use their influence to induce public officials to consult with them as a group on matters of public health. This was a symbiotic relationship necessary for medical advancement. America – and Philadelphia in particular – owes Edinburgh much for developing a model of medical organisation that was largely, though not entirely, exportable.[9]

Comparing the roster of the first faculty of the medical school with that of the founding senior Fellows of the College, four names reappear: Morgan, Rush, Shippen, and Kuhn. Each was taught by Cullen, and a closer look at the careers of these notable Americans can tell us something about Cullen's influence on American medicine.

Morgan founded the medical school at 'Penn', and Rush was the motive force behind the creation of the College. Both were apprenticed to John Redman (1722–1808), the first president of the College of Physicians. Redman was born in Philadelphia. After graduating from the Presbyterian Log College at Nashaminy, he studied medicine under Dr John Kearsley who had come to Philadelphia from England in 1711 and who, as an Anglican, broke the virtual medical monopoly exercised by the Welsh Quakers in that town. Kearsley gathered about him a coterie of able students; John Redman was his most famous. Redman was among the first Philadelphians to go abroad for medical training. Following his apprenticeship to Kearsley around 1743, he practised medicine in Bermuda and then enrolled at Edinburgh University in October 1746, nine years before Cullen's arrival. He attended the lectures of Monro *primus* and those of Charles Alston, and spent the next year at Leiden, where he graduated. He returned to Philadelphia in 1749 (he lived two blocks from the College's first residence) and established one of the largest practices in the City. A large practice demanded apprentices, and Redman's included Morgan, Rush, Shippen the younger, and Wistar, all of whom he was able to commend to Edinburgh.

When the precocious John Morgan (see Figure 30, p43) arrived in Edinburgh in 1761, his intellectual baggage included more medical experience than any previous American student had brought with him. His father had emigrated from Wales as a Quaker, and had become very wealthy and very Anglican. Morgan completed his studies at a private school and spent six years in Philadelphia as Redman's apprentice. During that time he received his Bachelor of Arts degree with the College of Philadelphia's first graduating class in 1757, and later graduated Master of Arts there. He then served with lieutenant's rank as a military surgeon. In 1760 he travelled to London where he studied under William Hunter. Recommended to Cullen and Cullen's patron Lord Kames by Benjamin Franklin, Morgan won Cullen's enduring friendship. After leaving Edinburgh, Morgan settled in Paris, before embarking upon a grand tour – *un très grand tour* – that included an audience with Pope Clement XIII, a visit to Voltaire, a meeting with Morgagni, and the acquisition of a trunkful of licences and memberships, including a nomination for membership of the Royal College of Physicians of Edinburgh, and dozens of endorsements from influential patrons and scientists[10]. Handsome, cultured, wealthy, well educated, and superbly connected, he became 'the darling of the European profession', where his reputation as a notable American was second only to that of Franklin.[11]

Morgan visited other medical schools in Europe not just to round out his education; he actually became an advocate and emissary of Edinburgh's system on the Continent. Resisting the temptation of many offers to remain abroad, he wrote from London in November 1764 to Cullen, his close adviser, about his desire to return to Philadelphia to give medical lectures. When he returned to Philadelphia a few months later, he was equipped with a letter from Pennsylvania's proprietary Thomas Penn endorsing the founding of a medical school in Philadelphia, a letter which Morgan presented to the trustees of the College of Philadelphia along with a plan for the development and design of a medical school attached to the College. He requested an appointment as professor of medicine. On May 3, 1765, the trustees granted Morgan's request, elected him professor of the theory and practice of physic, and permitted him to deliver the College's commencement address at the end of the month. Morgan's address, his famous *Discourse upon the Institution of Medical Schools in America*, remains a classic.

Arguing for the need to regulate the practice of physic and to organise medical knowledge into specialised branches of study, he urged the pedagogical and practical separation of physic, surgery, and pharmacy. He proposed to institutionalise the natural branches of medical science – the theory and practice of medicine, anatomy, materia medica, botany, and chemistry – by appointing 'a coalition of able men, who would undertake to give compleat and regular courses of lectures' in each of these areas. Morgan would teach the practice of medicine and Shippen anatomy; in 1768 Kuhn was appointed professor of botany and materia medica; in 1769, Rush joined the faculty as professor of chemistry. Importantly, in 1766, Dr Thomas Bond (1712–84), the driving force behind the founding of the Pennsylvania Hospital in 1752, persuaded the Hospital's managers to allow its staff to offer clinical lectures at the medical school. In 1767, the medical school's trustees established requirements for matriculation and graduation that closely paralleled those of the University of Edinburgh, which was understandably viewed at the time as the College's parent institution. New York City emulated Philadelphia in short order. In 1771 the Philadelphia school awarded its first four doctoral degrees. About the only innovation that Morgan did not import from Edinburgh was his introduction to America of the practical superiority of the umbrella to the gold-headed cane.[12]

Writing from Edinburgh to Philadelphia in November 1766, Benjamin Rush (Figure 31, p44), the other of Redman's two most renowned 'professional children', declared to Morgan, who called Cullen the Boerhaave of his age, that Dr Cullen was wont to hold Morgan's accomplishments aloft as an encouragement to other American students.[13] Rush needed no further encouragement than the example of Cullen himself. Following five years of academic preparation at a Presbyterian boarding school, Rush, who was descended from English Quakers, entered the College of New Jersey, as Princeton was then called, and graduated a year and a half later in 1760 at the age of fifteen. He spent the next five and a half years as Redman's apprentice, during which time he attended the anatomy lectures of William Shippen, Jr. (Figure 32, p45), who had just returned from Edinburgh with his doctoral diploma and who later became a Fellow of the Royal College of Physicians. Rush also enrolled in Morgan's courses at the new medical school. Anticipating acute competition in the rapidly professionalising medical environment of Philadelphia, he was encouraged by his teachers to enroll in Edinburgh, where he became a disciple and friend of Cullen just two months before Cullen succeeded to the chair of the institutes of medicine.[14]

'*Dr. Cullen*', wrote Rush to Morgan in 1768, 'the great unrivalled *Dr. Cullen* is going on unfolding each Day some new facet to us in the Animal Oeconomy . . . I think I would not fail of having heard them [his lectures] for ten thousand pounds. [I]llustrious Oracle of human Wisdom live – live forever!'[15] Having obtained his doctor's degree in 1768 and hoping to 'be able to transplant most of his [Cullen's] Doctrines to Philadelphia', Rush returned home in 1769 and immediately started a practice.[16] He also began his tenure as the first professor of chemistry at the College of Philadelphia, where he taught a course that would have been quite familiar to Americans who had preceded him in Edinburgh.

Reflecting on Cullen's career, Rush praised his mentor as a teacher for his intelligibility, modesty, warmth, patience and encouragement of the values of scepticism and self-reliance. 'His constant aim', declared Rush, 'was to produce in their [his students'] minds a change from a passive to an active state; and to force upon them such habits of thinking, and observation, as should enable them to instruct themselves'. Rush recalled that, while lecturing about Galen in his course on the institutes of medicine in 1766, Cullen paused to declare: 'It is a great disadvantage to any science to have been improved by a great man. His authority imposes indolence, timidity, or idolatry upon all who come after him'.[17]

Ironically, as one of Cullen's American pupils confirmed to Rush in 1785, the students to whom Cullen administered heroic dosages of Enlightenment scepticism indeed idolised him.[18] Arriving in Edinburgh in October 1771 with letters of introduction from Rush and Morgan to the 'shining Oracle of Physic', Thomas Parke proceeded to take more than eleven hundred pages of manuscript notes from Cullen's lectures over the next seven months.[19] Adam Kuhn (Figure 33, p46) apparently did not merely take notes; he regurgitated them. Born in Philadelphia and trained in botany by Linnaeus (who named a plant after him), Kuhn received his MD degree in Edinburgh in 1767 and returned to Philadelphia the following year, when he was appointed professor of materia medica and botany at the College of Philadelphia. One of Kuhn's students regretted that his course contained no original ideas. 'From beginning to end', wrote Charles Caldwell, 'it was in substance but a transcript from the writings of Cullen'. According to Kuhn, that fact legitimated his course.[20] Philip Syng Physick, who received his MD degree from Edinburgh in 1792 and came to occupy the first chair in surgery at the University of Pennsylvania, began his medical studies with Kuhn by memorising Cullen's entire *First Lines*.[21] Obviously, Cullen's impact was huge; but was his influence lasting? Rush proclaimed that, by teaching 'the art of teaching' to the eventual professors at the Medical School of the University of Pennsylvania, Cullen 'had conveyed the benefits of his discoveries into every part of the United States.[22] What were those discoveries? And what were their purported benefits?

My predecessors at this lectern have made eloquently and abundantly clear at this symposium and in their published writings that it is difficult to extrapolate a neat relationship between theory and practice. Morgan assimilated Cullen's teachings and practised relatively moderate medicine. Rush assimilated Cullen's teachings and devised an heroic regimen that William Cobbett called 'one of those great discoveries which are made from time to time for the depopulation of the earth'.[23] In fact, as Professor Risse has persuasively shown by examining the therapeutic recommendations made by Cullen as a consultant, Cullen could maintain his roles as systematic theorist and eclectic practitioner without much cognitive dissonance.[24] Americans had little trouble doing the same. The picture is further clouded because, though Cullen was a thoughtful system builder, he was, as Professors Bynum and Risse have convincingly argued, a contingent rather than an essentialist nosologist. He intended his system to be heuristic.[25] Accordingly, he revised his views over a period that extended beyond the brief exposures to them of his cisatlantic pupils. We must also keep in mind that what one chooses to impart and what another chooses or happens to learn are seldom the same, and that the transcription and recopying of lecture notes inevitably increased the noise-to-signal ratio of communication. It is ironic but not suprising that Cullen's medical system, as Dr Risse has pointed out, became quickly forgotten shortly after his death in 1790.[26]

No, contrary to Rush's eulogistic claim, Cullen did not extend his discoveries by teaching Americans the art of teaching. Rather, the imaginative cultivation of the art of teaching was Cullen's discovery as well as his most precious gift to those who sought to extend the benefits of the finest medical education to be found anywhere in the world. His insistence on lecturing in English rather than Latin, his ability to shape his courses to meet the needs, backgrounds, and capacities of his pupils, his superb expository style and sharply critical outlook account for his deserved popularity and enduring legacy.[27] Cullen's influence is too often associated with his system. Professor Risse's careful research has shown that Cullen 'was by far the most outspoken and skeptical teacher visiting the infirmary'. Systems to him were merely 'temporary platforms from which to view the evidence and gather new facts . . .' Cullen taught his students that 'What ultimately mattered was the direct clinical experience as the *only* guide to diagnostic judgements and therapeutic indications'. These viewpoints persisted long after his system became obsolete. As values and methods, they constituted vehicles for the dissemination and analysis of newer ideas and discoveries.

Cullen, then, was a teacher with a persuasive pedagogy and warm personality who befriended many of his American pupils and who influenced them by force of example. He also was a 'great man' whose testimonial could help establish the career of an ambitious novitiate.[28] He developed a model of clinical teaching and a style of professional conduct which were deliberately and at times unconsciously replicated in North America and assimilated by individuals who never left the first new nation for training abroad. He wrote books and lectures which – authorised or pirated or transcribed from notes and memory – served as the sacramentals of American medical schooling and as texts against which Americans could refine their opaque perspectives. As a scientist, clinician, theorist, organisational strategist, teacher, friend and academic politician – indeed as all the things my distinguished predecessors at this lectern have so well examined – Cullen's direct and indirect influence was indeed considerable.

Many of the Fellows of the College of Physicians of Philadelphia who had marched in the funeral procession for Benjamin Franklin less than three months earlier, convened at the College on July 9, 1790, for a memorial service to William Cullen. Six years before, Cullen had sent his 'respectful and affectionate compliments to all my old pupils at Philadelphia. I shall always hold it my highest honour that the founders of the Medical College of Philadelphia were all of them my Pupils and if it can be known I think it will be the most certain means of transmitting my name to a distant posterity for I believe that this School will one day or other be the greatest in the world'. The entire medical community was invited to the service, and among the attendees were several of

Cullen's old pupils.[29] Undoubtedly, Cullen represented intellectual and institutional contributions which were greater than his own individual achievements. But, as Rush's eulogy makes clear, his own achievements were extraordinary. His established eminence at Edinburgh garnered him a reputation which drew to him students who might otherwise not have assimilated those larger contributions so quickly or so thoroughly.

American historians of medicine seem generally to have over-estimated what John Harley Warner calls the eighteenth century's 'spirit of system' and to have associated too closely Cullen's influence with this phenomenon in order, perhaps, to glorify the nineteenth century's revolt against systems. Thus, they have simplified and distorted Cullen's legacy. Indeed when one looks at the debates taking place among the early Fellowship of the College of Physicians of Philadelphia, one encounters exactly the kind of critical discourse Cullen successfully stimulated in Edinburgh. Two hundred years after Cullen's death, many of the College's purposes have changed decisively. It now endeavours, among other goals, to serve as a chief repository and interpreter of American medical history. And, as its Fellows long ago learned so much of medicine from Cullen and Edinburgh, so today it continues to learn much from Edinburgh about medicine's history.

Acknowledgements

The author wishes to thank Thomas A. Horrocks, Director of the Library for Historical Services, College of Physicians of Philadelphia, and his staff for guidance to the proper sources; Whitfield J. Bell Jr, for being such an exhaustive source of knowledge and reliable interpreter of colonial American medicine; and, Nancy J. Tomes, Acting Director of the F.C. Wood Institute for the History of Medicine, College of Physicians of Philadelphia, for kindly reviewing this text.

Notes and references

1. W. James, *The Varieties of Religious Experience* (London: Longmans, Green, and Co., 1902), p.1.
2. See, for example, W.J. Bell Jr, 'A Portrait of the Colonial Physician', *Bull. Hist. of Med.* 44 (1970): 497–517.
3. Samuel Bard to John Bard, Edinburgh, 4 Feb. 1764, Bard Collection, N.Y. Acad. Med; quoted in W.J. Bell, Jr, 'Some American Students of "that Shining Oracle of Physic" Dr. William Cullen of Edinburgh, 1755–1766', *Proc. Amer. Phil. Soc.* 94 (1950): 275.
4. C. and J. Bridenbaugh, *Rebels and Gentlemen: Philadelphia in the Age of Franklin* (London: Oxford Univ. Press, 1962), pp. 3–4, 293; M. Kraus, *The Atlantic Civilization: Eighteenth Century Origins*, (N.Y: Cornell Univ. Press, 1949).
5. R.H. Girdwood, 'The Influence of Scotland on North American Medicine', in *The Influence of Scottish Medicine: An Historical Assessment of Its International Impact*, ed. D.A. Dow (Carnforth, England: The Parthenon Publishing Group, 1988), pp. 31–42; W.J. Bell, Jr, *The Colonial Physician & Other Essays* (N.Y: Science History Publications,

1975), p. 42; R.H. Shryock, *The Development of Modern Medicine* (N.Y: Alfred A. Kropf, 1936) p.43.

6. Thomas Ruston, holograph petition, Edinburgh, 17 April 1764, in Thomas Ruston Papers, Historical Collections, College of Physicians of Philadelphia; Adam Smith to William Cullen, 20 September 1774, in The *Correspondence of Adam Smith*, quoted in J.V. Golinski, 'Utility and Audience in Eighteenth-Century Chemistry: Case Studies of William Cullen and Joseph Priestly', *Br. J. Hist. Sci.* 21 (1988): 15.

7. W.J. Bell Jr, *The College of Physicians of Philadelphia: A Bicentennial History* (Canton, MA: Science History Publications, U.S.A., 1987), p. 9; Bell, note 5 above, p. 41; R.S. Klein, 'Dr. George Glentworth (1735–1792): A Physician Eminent and Useful', *Trans. & Studies Coll. Physicians Philadelphia* 34 (1966–7): 117–20; W.S. Middleton, 'Samuel Powel Griffitts', *Ann. Med. Hist.* 10 (1938): 474–90.

8. J.H. Cassedy, 'Medicine and the Learned Society in the United States, 1660–1850', in *The Pursuit of Knowledge in the Early American Republic: American Scientific and Learned Societies from Colonial Times to the Civil War*, ed. A. Oleson and S.C. Brown (Baltimore: The Johns Hopkins Univ. Press, 1976), p. 261; W.G. Rothstein, *American Physicians in the Nineteenth Century: From Sects to Science* (Baltimore: The Johns Hopkins Univ. Press, 1972), pp. 63–6.

9. In his marvellous history of the College of Physicians of Philadelphia published in 1987 on the occasion of the College's bicentennial celebration, Whitfield Bell cautions astutely against the filiopietistic tendency to assume the College of Physicians of Philadelphia is a lineal descendant of either the Royal College of London or the Royal College of Edinburgh (Bell, note 7 above, p.10). Dr Bell's point is indisputable. Considering, however, the facts that the College of Physicians of Philadelphia was presided over by Edinburgh-trained physicians for its first half century of existence and that I am delivering this humble paper within the hallowed walls of the Royal College, I would beg Dr Bell for a bit of historiographic flexibility on this issue. Of course, should I be alive and sufficiently fortunate to be invited to the Royal College of London's semi-millenial celebration, I should like to reserve the right to revisionism.

10. Bridenbaugh and Bridenbaugh, note 4 above, pp. 264–69; Bell, note 5 above, pp. 194–204.

11. W.J. Bell Jr, *John Morgan, Continental Doctor* (Philadelphia: Univ. of Pennsylvania Press, 1965), pp. 54–99; Bridenbaugh and Bridenbaugh, note 4 above, p. 248.

12. F.R. Packard, 'How London and Edinburgh Influenced Medicine in Philadelphia in the Eighteenth Century', *Trans. Coll. Physicians Philadelphia* 53 (1931): 164–67; J. Duffy, *The Healers: A History of American Medicine* (Chicago Univ. of Illinois Press, 1976), pp. 63–5; Bridenbaugh and Bridenbaugh, note 4 above, pp. 285–9.

13. Rush to Morgan, Edinburgh 16 November 1766, Gratz Collection, Historical Society of Pennsylvania, cited in Bell, note 5 above, p. 59.

14. N.G. Goodman, *Benjamin Rush: Physician and Citizen, 1746–1813* (Philadelphia: Univ. of Pennsylvania Press, 1934), pp. 8–32.

15. Rush to Morgan, Edinburgh, 27 July 1768, in Joseph Carson, 'History of the Medical Department of the University of Pennsylvania' (MS Scrapbook, College of Physicians of Philadelphia), II. p.27.

16. Rush to Morgan, Edinburgh, 20 January 1768, in *ibid.*, II, p. 23.

17. Rush, *An Eulogium in Honor of the Late Dr. William Cullen, Professor of the Practice of Physic in the University of Edinburgh; delivered before the College of Physicians of Philadelphia, on the 9th of July, agreeably to their Vote on the 4th of May, 1790* (Philadelphia: Thomas Dobson, 1790), pp. 12–17, 28.

18. J.R.B. Rodgers to Rush, Edinburgh, 20 July 1785, Rush MSS (Library Company of Philadelphia, Ridgway Branch), cited in Bell, note 5 above, p. 54.
19. Bell, note 5 above, p. 77.
20. M.E. Brown, 'Adam Kuhn: Eighteenth Century Physician and Teacher', *J. Hist. Med. Allied Sci.* 5 (1950): pp. 163–77, esp. pp. 167–9; C. Caldwell, *Autobiography*, ed. H.W. Warner (Philadelphia: Lippincott, 1855), p. 124.
21. Bell, note 5 above, p. 44.
22. Rush, note 17 above, p. 23.
23. R.H. Shryock, *Medicine and Society in America: 1660–1860* (N.Y: Cornell University Press, 1960), pp. 67–70; William Cobbett, In *The Rush Light* (N.Y: 28 February, 1800), p. 49.
24. G.B. Risse, '"Doctor William Cullen, Physician, Edinburgh": A Consultation Practice in the Eighteenth Century', *Bull. Hist. Med.* 48 (1974): 338–51.
25. W.F. Bynum, 'Cullen and the Study of Fevers in Britain, 1760–1820', *Medical History*, Supplement No. 1 (1981): pp. 135–147; G.B. Risse, *Hospital Life in Enlightenment Scotland: Care and Teaching at the Royal Infirmary of Edinburgh* (Cambridge: Cambridge Univ. Press, 1986), p. 278.
26. Risse, *ibid*. pp. 260, 278; Risse, note 24 above, p. 339.
27. J.K. Crellin, 'William Cullen: his Calibre as a Teacher, and an Unpublished Introduction to his *A Treatise of the Materia Medica*, London, 1773', *Medical History*, 15 (1971): pp. 79–87; R. Stott, 'William Cullen and Edinburgh Medicine: a Re-appraisal', *Soc. Social Hist. Med. Bull.* 38 (1986): 7–9.
28. Deprived of study abroad or a recommendation from Cullen, one could at least alter one's name, as did Elisha Dick of Marcus Hook, Pennsylvania, who, upon initiating medical studies, adopted the middle name of Cullen; J.M. Turner, 'Sketch of the Life of Elisha Cullen Dick', *Trans. Med. Soc. Virginia* (1883–5), pp. 270–71.
29. Cullen to Rush, Edinburgh, 16 October 1784, Rush MSS (Library Company of Philadelphia. Ridgway), XXIV, 56; quoted in Bell, note 5 above, p. 59; Bell, note 7 above, p. 16.

The first forty years of the Royal Medical Society and the part William Cullen played in it*

DONALD C. MACARTHUR

The Medical Society of Edinburgh was formally constituted in 1737 and granted a Royal Charter in 1778. It is one of the oldest medical societies in Europe. Founded in an era when enthusiasm for knowledge and debate knew no bounds, the Society provided a forum for public speaking and dialectic amongst the students of the developing medical school in the city, and was a model for many of the other debating societies to appear in Edinburgh during the Scottish Enlightenment of the close of the eighteenth century. Two and a half centuries later, having had to move with the years both in terms of outlook and location, the Society is still thriving. The ideals of its founders and early members having been maintained, the Society recognises its considerable debt to these men of great character and conviction – men such as William Cullen who contributed to the Society as a student, as a celebrated teacher, physician and honorary member and as a professor in the University of Edinburgh.

The origins of the Society can be traced to August 1734 when an offer was made to Dr Alexander Russell 'for a pecuniary gratification of the body of a young woman, a stranger, just then dead by a fever of ten days' standing'. Russell and five others (Dr George Cleghorn, Dr William Cumming, Mr Alexander Hamilton, Dr James Kennedy and Dr Archibald Taylor) dissected the body over the next months in the anatomical theatre, the use of which had been readily granted to them by Alexander Monro *primus* on the application of Cumming. On completing the dissection the group spent what they described as 'a social evening at a tavern' during which Taylor proposed that they should continue to meet fortnightly within their lodgings, taking it in turn to prepare and read a dissertation on some medical subject. Cumming was unfortunate enough during the dissection to have been

---

*The speech at the symposium dinner, held in the rooms of the Royal Medical Society, made by the Society's Senior President before proposing a toast to the Memory of William Cullen.

afflicted with the same fever as had been responsible for the provision of the cadaver, but he survived and at the first such meeting presented a dissertation on 'The signs, causes and methods of cure of the *Rabies Canina*'. The six went on to meet throughout the winter and spring, but in the summer of 1735 they dispersed, with Cleghorn alone remaining in Edinburgh.

In the autumn of 1735, George Cleghorn along with Dr John Fothergill and a number of others resumed similar meetings. Amongst the students attending these meetings was William Cullen, who spent the winter sessions of 1734–5 and 1735–6 attending medical classes in Edinburgh prior to starting practice in Hamilton. Many years later Cullen wrote to a friend, 'Your uncle and I are, I believe, the only surviving members of a society which existed at Edinburgh in the year 1735 and which laid the foundation of the Medical Society . . . tell your worthy uncle that I have . . . a manuscript book in which the discourses of the society in 1735 are recorded; and there are I believe some of his juvenile performances to be found in it'.

The first formal constitution of the Society came in 1737, with its code of laws describing it as 'a society instituted at Edinburgh for Improvement in Medical Knowledge'. It was from this date that an accurate roll of members was kept. One of the ten members of the original session was Stuart Threipland, an ardent Jacobite who spent the months leading up to Culloden with Prince Charles, the Stuart Pretender; surviving the battle, Threipland went into hiding before fleeing to France. On returning to practise in Edinburgh in 1747, Threipland went on to become President of the Royal College of Physicians. Another of the ten was James Russell, later professor of natural philosophy at Edinburgh. Other notable characters who were members of the Society during its first few sessions were Francis Home (who later became the first professor of materia medica at Edinburgh), Mark Akenside (later physician to the Queen), John Roebuck (who founded the Carron Iron Company), John Hope (the great botanist) and Richard Brocklesby (later a physician of eminence in London).

Initially meetings were held once a week in a tavern in the vicinity of the University, with a president being appointed each week to conduct the proceedings. These consisted of a discourse on a medical subject by a member, consideration of a case of a disease, discussion of an important medical question and then debate over an Aphorism of Hippocrates. The form of the meetings was therefore similar to that of the examination for the degree of Doctor of Medicine which was then awarded on the completion of undergraduate studies. Membership in the early years was somewhat exclusive and considered a great honour, since it only took a single negative for a petition for a seat to be rejected. Debate was spirited and reflected both the teachings of the professors and opposition to many of their ideas, which were considered by some to lay too much emphasis on the by now somewhat dated Boerhaavian system. Some time in the 1740s the managers of the new Royal Infirmary granted the Society permission to hold its meetings in a vacant room there and the funds that had previously paid for accommodation in a tavern began to be used to accumulate a library.

Clinical teaching had been introduced to Edinburgh by John Rutherford with a series of lectures in the Infirmary in the winter of 1746–7. Around this time, the Society's members set up a Clinical Board for the mutual benefit of their clinical experience and the sick poor. The first Obligation Book, in which members joining the Society signed their name reflects this in containing the detailed regulations for the care of patients by members.

In 1753, Oliver Goldsmith arrived in Edinburgh from Ireland to study medicine, tradition having it that he lodged alongside Joseph Black and Adam Ferguson in College Wynd (now Guthrie Street), at that time almost entirely populated by learned men and professors. Goldsmith joined the Medical Society in January 1753 but did not remain in Edinburgh long enough to read a dissertation. He was not enamoured with most of his teachers and even less so with Edinburgh's social life, but he made a great impact on his fellows as much by virtue of his wardrobe as his personality. Such, however, was the unbounded benevolence of his disposition that by 1754 he found himself in considerable debt and was forced to flee the country to avoid imprisonment.

William Cullen returned to Edinburgh in 1756 as joint professor of chemistry. In 1752 his student protégé Joseph Black had preceded him in moving from Glasgow to Edinburgh. Here Black completed his medical studies, and during this undergraduate period made his famous discovery of 'fixed air' or carbon dioxide. Black was elected an honorary member of the Medical Society in 1767 and his portrait was painted for the Society by David Martin in 1787. This is now on loan to the Scottish National Portrait Gallery, with a small copy hung in the Society's Meeting Hall.

By the 1760s the Society had some twenty to thirty members meeting every Saturday in the Royal Infirmary with meetings lasting about four hours, and there were four annually appointed Presidents. John Brown joined the Society in 1761 on turning from the study of Divinity to that of Medicine. Industrious and extremely well-read, he was noted for his cynical nature and considerable intemperance. It seems he was a popular man, since he was President on three occasions in the 1770s. The Brunonian theory of disease that he later developed stood in contrast to the rigorous classification of Cullen and was the subject of considerable debate in the ensuing years. Within the Medical Society at one point the convictions of the supporters of the two theories were so great that it was deemed necessary to pass a law which forbade duelling.

Cullen, who had been lecturing in clinical medicine since 1757 was increasing both in respect and popularity as a teacher amongst the Society's members, and in 1764 he was elected an honorary member. During his teaching life in Edinburgh he had maintained a strong interest in the activities of the Medical Society, the foundation of which he had helped to lay as a student. Nowhere was this more evident than in his involvement with the building of a new Hall for the Society.

The growth in numbers attending meetings and the expansion of a library which had thrived on increasing funds and a steady flow of presents from past members meant that the accommodation in the Royal Infirmary was no longer sufficient. It was clear that the Society would benefit from having a building of its own, and in 1771 a committee was formed to deal with this matter. It consisted of Dr Cullen, Dr John Gregory and the four Presidents, including six times President Dr Andrew Duncan senior, founder of the Public Dispensary and the Edinburgh Asylum for the Insane. A subscription list was opened and sufficient funds were on hand by 1775 to allow the Society to begin building a Hall. An area of ground was granted for the purpose by the College of Surgeons, close to their Hall, on the west side of Surgeons Square, adjoining what is now the Old High School. The site and plan of the building had been suggested by Cullen and he, along with several other members of the Faculty of Medicine, headed the subscription list. The foundation stone of the new Hall was laid on 21st April, 1775, by William Cullen during his presidency of the Royal College of Physicians. The ceremony was attended by the other medical professors and the whole of the Medical Society. Prior to the ceremony an extraordinary meeting was held in Surgeons' Hall at which an address was delivered by Gilbert Blane, one of the Presidents of the Society. Referring to the founders of the Society, Blane said that they had 'perceived, that it was in Society alone, by mutual communication and reflection of the lights of reason and knowledge, that the intellectual as well as the moral powers of man are exalted and perfected'. The dinner which followed the occasion is reported to have been an extremely cordial one, with Cullen giving a toast 'May the professors and students always live in amity together, and sometimes drink wine together'.

The Medical Hall was opened on 21st April 1776. It contained three large rooms, one to serve as a meeting hall, one as a repository for the, by now, valuable book collection and a third to be used for chemical experiments. Robert Freer, six times President, delivered the inaugural address extolling the generosity of those who had contributed to the building of the Hall.

In the space of barely forty years a society which had arisen through the friendship and enterprise of a small number of students had gained enough influence to finance the building of its own hall. The precipitous rise of the Society paralleled both the growth of the Medical School and the distinguished career of Cullen who had played such a great part in the development of both institutions.

The legacy of Cullen to the Medical Society did not end there. His sons Henry and Archibald were both members of the Society (Archibald a President in 1780), as were many of his eminent pupils such as William Withering (who established the medicinal value of foxglove) and Gilbert Blane (who was successful in persuading the Royal Navy to recognise the work of James Lind, and to introduce lemon juice for the prevention of scurvy).

When Cullen resigned his chair in 1789, the Society held a meeting of his pupils and admirers to determine a suitable memorial to his great services to medicine. A bust of him by William Gowan was placed in the new University buildings which were then being erected, and a portrait painted in 1776 by David Martin for the Medical Society is now on loan to the Scottish National Portrait Gallery, a copy of which hangs today beside a portrait of Joseph Black in the Society's Meeting Hall. The carved slab covering the foundation stone laid by Cullen in 1775 has been transferred to the Society's current rooms in the University Student Centre, and a silver medal which he had placed within the foundation stone is now the Senior President's badge of office.

These memorials ensure that the name of William Cullen, so influential throughout its early history, lives on in the minds of those who now constitute the Royal Medical Society.

My Lord, Ladies and Gentlemen, I give you a toast:

THE MEMORY OF WILLIAM CULLEN.

Index

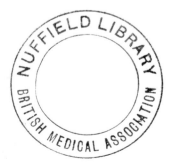